AWAKE!

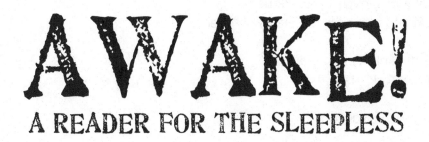

AWAKE!

A READER FOR THE SLEEPLESS

edited by
Steven Lee Beeber

SOFT SKULL PRESS
2008

Awake! A Reader For the Sleepless
Copyright © 2008 by Steven Lee Beeber
Editorial Matter All rights reserved under International and Pan-American
Copyright Conventions

Library of Congress Cataloging-in-Publication Data available from
the Library of Congress

Cover Design: Gary Fogelson
Interior Design: David Barnett
Printed in the United States of America

Soft Skull Press
New York, NY

www.softskull.com

ISBN-10 1-933368-79-9
ISBN-13 978-1-933368-79-5

I never sleep at night

But just the same

I never weep at night

"I Call Your Name" – The Beatles

TABLE OF CONTENTS

TUESDAY

WEDNESDAY

THURSDAY

FRIDAY

AWAKE!

SATURDAY

SUNDAY

WHO? HOW? HUH?

INTRODUCTION
Steven Lee Beeber

Consider the career of Vincent Spano. I have. Lying awake, my left cheek pressed to the scruff of the sofa, my eyes shiny with the jumping light of the TV, I've stared at him on screen and wondered, "How does he sleep at night? And when he doesn't, how can he face his movies?" You may not be familiar with them by name, but you've probably seen them—that is, if you've been awake late at night, unable to sleep and desperate for distraction, flipping through infomercials and *Girls Gone Wild* ads ("... now they're partying!!!") in search of something, anything, to take you out of yourself, the heavy *presence* of yourself, your body too hot or too soft or too itchy ("Get me some air in here!" "Why don't I go to the gym?!" "Damn these infernal mosquitoes!"), your mind working almost physically behind your skull, a pressure in league with your heart, the beating one and the figurative one, a throbbing that is also a numbing—*gotta get to sleep, gotta get up, gotta get to sleep so I can get up*—the rump-a-bum-bum hypnotic mania of *can't do what you wanna do what you need to do* everything up-downwards, the exhaustion of being awake itself seeming to keep you awake, the *awakeawakeawakefuckthis* mantra of *relaxrelaxrelax* at its tail end, push me and pull you, pushes me, pulls you, tears apart, like love, but no, you're still awake, no break, no drop ...

Yes, when I'm like this, I consider the career of Vincent Spano.

Don't get me wrong. It's not as if Spano is that bad. He's adequate. You can watch him in a film and for the vast majority of it not think, "I'm watching a film; that is someone acting there; there's a camera on that street that I can't see photographing him, and everyone else is acting, too; this all fake and not just real life playing out." The suspension of disbelief and all that. You can do it with his films, basically. But they'll never move you. They'll never carry you. They'll never show you a different life in its particulars, its essence, as you would otherwise not have seen it. They'll never make something about LIFE shine forth for you in such a way that you mutter under your breath, "Yes, it's like that. Like that for me. Yes. And for you." Not with Vincent Spano. Not with his too basic skills. His unimpressive skills. His talents, adequate at best, but little more. No, he won't do it for you. And he knows that he won't. And that's what's worst. The ultimate curse. The human condition of awareness. It's bad when you know you're bad. Or just adequate. Nothing special. Another blob on the planet, taking your water balloon of skin-and-blood upstairs and over grocery store floors and down to auditions, knowing that if you disappeared nothing would really change, and in the general sense, it would clearly not matter. You know this and you hate this and you feel your check pressing into the couch, your eyes dry and warming, your thirst insistent, but you don't want to get up, you don't have the energy to get up, you're exhausted, no rest, exhausted and you've had enough of this, exhausted staring at Vincent on two channels, back and forth and back and forth, and it's equally bad, your flab, your belly, your sweating crotch in your boxers beneath the blanket, bad, nothing feels right, exhausted and far too awakeawakeawake, and nothing to do but look, see, dwell on things in the middle of the night, almost the morning, the what-is-it hour, the too-late-to-sleep-before-work-anyway hour . . . too early to get up for work really . . . too too too too . . .

Fuck!

You know about this, right? You've been there? Surely I am not alone? For clearly there are others out there who experience much the same. Oh, I don't mean that they consider the career of Vincent Spano (though I wouldn't be surprised if there are a few who do. There are always a few somewhere, some time, doing much the same as you are doing). No, it's more that I am joined in my sleeplessness, my restlessness, my insomnia. I mean, look at the ads that come on between those Vincent Spano movies:

"Are you looking for a good night's rest?"

Yes!

"Do you find yourself exhausted upon waking?"

Indeed!

"Wouldn't you be happier with Ambient in your life?"

Sure, why not!

"Ambient: side effects include constipation, resignation and loss of memory."

Shit!

Yes, there are many others out there doing much as I at the same time in their separate places. They are lying awake, just as they have countless times before. Just as I have from almost as far back as I can remember, the heartbeat sound of the radiator kicking in behind the walls, making me feel that the whole house was alive in some sense as I lay there, going back over my thoughts up to that moment. "I heard the heartbeat sound while I was thinking about the Lone Ranger's pal, Tonto, and I thought of Tonto because of my friend Alex Wolinsky, and Alex entered my head because I was thinking about school and recess and how we do different things on days when it rains than when it's sunny . . ."

And on and on as far as I could go, long into the night, a backwards trail of breadcrumbs to wherever I'd "started."

It wasn't much different in high school, either—in terms of not sleeping, that is—though by then I wasn't passively lying in bed but up at my desk under lamplight with my headphones on, listening to "I'm So Tired" or "I Am the Walrus" as I sketched out poem after poem that I knew would one day make my name:

I bite off my thumb and begin to laugh
Bloody flesh between my teeth
And spitting it into the gutter, I run.

and

Men with Swiss cheese skin
the holes scream and stare
the nightmare resistance of existence makes them laugh
ha ha ha ha ha . . .

Ha ha ha ha indeed.

It seems funny now, but in many ways I was dead serious then. Dead seriously awake, that is. Dead seriously up for most of the night. Rationalizing it with the proud disclaimer "Sleep is Stupid," saying that in chemistry class the next morning, my hair coarse from the hottest showers I could take, my eyes probably glazed and a bit frightening to my classmates.

"Do you know that you lose a third of your life unconscious in sleep?"

"I like sleeping," Katy Schwebin says. "I like to dream."

"I like to dream of sleeping with you," smirks Fred Seagan.

Laughter all around. While my eyes itched. And my mouth felt pasty and white.

15

AWAKE!

By college I was *using* this lack of rest, pulling all-nighters when all-nighters weren't necessary, doodling in my notebook if I'd already done my work. Or writing the first of my "adult-era" short stories. Oedipal parables of kids in love with their Daisy (as in Gatsby) Duck cocoa cups; memories of a Southern-Jewish Seder (a certain relative designated "redneckus judaicus" in nomenclature); a strange piece that I actually still like that began with the phrase, "I have a bad attitude, and it's a good thing," though that little darling was ultimately cut in the final script.

Yes, all this sleeplessness. Sleeplessness well into my first job at a weekly newspaper, out at the bars till 4 a.m. (when they closed), into the office at 6 a.m. before anyone else showed up (aside from the electronic typesetter, a disgruntled-employee-looking wisp of thinning hair dubbed "the weasel"), banging out 1500-word pieces in a blaze of adrenaline and crystal meth, features about attending a nudist colony on "Las Vegas Night" ("The Naked and the Nude") or riding with the garbage men on their rounds through the wealthiest suburb in the city ("Rich White Trash") or heading out with the repo man the week before Christmas ("the Anti-Claus taketh away thy wheels"). These and many other pieces. And would I have done them, had I slept? Would I have had the energy or presence of body to use my time in this way? I don't know for sure. After all, I was never able, as scientists say, to "run the control." I only lived one life, not its alternatives.

Today, a decade or so on, I'm still waking after an hour or two of sleep, still meeting the dawn with a scowl and a stare, still occasionally feeling that surge of caffeine-like energy as I head out long before most, waiting at the door of Starbucks as the "barista" unlocks it, asking for my "grande" in such a way that I unnerve myself, not having spoken in hours despite all the activity inside. Taking that mug and sitting down with my computer and doing the laptop dance of Beethoven at his keyboard, typing so rapidly, so fluidly, so easily that I think sometimes, "Sleep is for losers. It's stupid!"

So you see, we never really do leave high school. And we never really grow out of who we are. Even if we modify the product and offer new and improved versions.

And perhaps that's part of what drives us to insomnia. That awareness, that consciousness, that sense of knowing too much about ourselves and our world. Like Vincent Spano. The human condition. The actor's condition. The Spano Complex. The Vincent Spano Syndrome. What have you.

16

In putting together this anthology, I wanted to learn a bit more about what my fellow sufferers (or is that chosen few?) were doing in their own late night hours. Their midnight confessions were what I wanted to hear. Their after-hours tales. Those things that you only tell the four walls.

And then too I really just wanted to create something to aid others as they lay awake, UN-asleep. As they lay there trying to drift off, phase out, blank the mind, descend once again, back down back down back down. I wanted to give them an alternative. Something other than a movie or a book unrelated to what they were feeling. I wanted to give them a gift of gab. All these writers-artists-poets-and-the-rest giving voice to their own experiences of insomnia, their own sense of what it means to be awake, their own alternative universes in the night. Not a cure, you see, but an evocation, a shared experience, a place to feel at peace, if not at rest.

And so I hope this provides for you as well. Because those hours alone when the world is asleep can be lonely ones. Or scattered ones. Or painful ones. And then, at other times, they can be giddy ones, manic ones, riotous ones. They have many sides and many facets and many ways of being. Both mine and yours and theirs and the rest. And Vincent Spano's too. Wherever he is. Watching his movies. Thinking about his past. Awake.

So welcome, dear reader. Flip through these pages. And do not go gentle into that good night.

SUNDAY

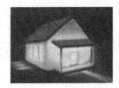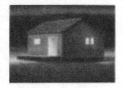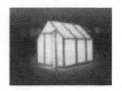

Sleep Won't Come

THOUGHTS ENTERTAINED WHILE ATTEMPTING TO SLEEP
FRANZ WRIGHT

1. POPULATION

The whole city could go in the time it takes a struck match to ignite

In the eyes of the old man who bitterly sold me my newspaper each day

I saw

In the hospital lights flickering all night through the park through the leaves of black wind

On things about to disappear who's closed his eyes in time?

And the little white candle of morphine the slightest of breaths could put out, so many

Startled, intaken

Breath

2. Old Man at Work at a School Child's Desk

Ecstasy of the sun, of perceiving
the sun, lost in childhood and only regained
in the word sun
and then
some decades later

in the sun.

ILLUSIVE BITCH
LYDIA LUNCH

I love Sleep, that illusive bitch, but Sleep hates me. Just the way it is. I can't se-
duce her into tolerating me for more than a few hours a night. Fickle cunt. Oh . . .
she'll allow me into her warm embrace. Five minutes after my head hits the pillows,
I'll be swimming into a delicious nocturnal numbness. But before R.E.M. has a chance
to cock his nugget against mine, Sleep, that fricking creep, screams for her night
nurse Insomnia to kick me in the head like a bouncer at a funeral party, and faster
than you can say THE QUICK AND THE DEAD, I no longer am. Asleep that is. Bitch.

I've tried over-the-counter as well as various prescribed medications, including,
but not limited to: Klonopin, Ativan, Halcion, Xanax, Valium, Melatonin, Marihuana,
Valerian Root, and Heroin. I've tortured myself with exhaustive workouts followed
by a hot bath preceding tantric sex where I practiced deep breathing in conjunction
with meditation and visualization techniques.

I gave up nicotine, sugar, spice, and tried a light box. Didn't help. I quit coffee.
HA! Anyone who has suffered from decades-long Insomnia knows damn well that
that ain't gonna last. You are going to need all the caffeine you can suck down in
order to function above that semi-somnambulant state of dream-deprived Sleep
that results in a numb narcosis, a permanent twilight zone, rarely fully conscious,
never completely asleep. Exhausted, but jacked up, like an electric rigor mortis that
short circuits the neurotransmitters creating a dense fog of chronic irritation that
can cloud even the simplest of tasks.

I am not referring to a few nights or even months of unfit Sleep, the youthful
buzz of which invigorates the blood stream, rife with recollections of uncountable
naughty deeds performed under the influence of designer cocktails. No, this miserable
ditty is a song of the sirens to the janitors of lunacy who have certainly not made
peace, for there is none to be made, after nearly half a century of stalking Morpheus,
that cruel trickster who only grants the occasional performance, and then upon a
stage so soaked with blood and guts that the sheer magnitude of his insane cruelty
creates a magnificent terror from which one is throttled awake, soaked in sweat,

choked by tears and stifling a scream, which unleashed would wake the very dead themselves, those lucky bastards to whom sleep is an eternal given.

Even in the cradle, I couldn't Sleep. I can recollect conversations I was too young to decipher. The winning hand held by my father on a typical Friday night poker marathon. The date the gas bill was due. Useless drivel. I started Sleepwalking at six. Talking to the electrical sockets in the living room. Directing traffic in my pajamas. Urinating in the refrigerator. Suffocating my younger brother with a ratty teddy bear. By the age of nine, already terminally Sleep-deprived, my nightmares were so gruesome that horror films read like bad comedies to my twisted pre-adolescent psyche.

Youth feeds on adrenaline. Who needs Sleep when you're a rambunctious teenager carousing through the night gallery of new experience? Or a rampaging twenty-something hellbent on accomplishing as much as possible, living life to the fullest, glutting on potential and wilding in the streets desperate to make your mark before that grump Thanatos comes a-calling. And what the hell . . . I'LL SLEEP WHEN I'M DEAD becomes the young psychos' mantra screamed into the crack of an unforgiving Dawn who is always able to creep up upon you faster than you could ever dream of outrunning her.

For most of my life I just didn't NEED more than four hours of Sleep a night. I felt great, I glowed, got a shitload of work done, loved the twilight hours between 3 and 6 a.m. when the rest of the world died or at least wasn't crawling up my ass with its noise, its complaints, its problems and demands. But enough is enough; or let me rephrase that: now there just ISN'T enough. Ever. I am jolted awake after a three-hour stint kissing Slumber. Doesn't matter how exhausted, drained or in pain. And PAIN happens. Migraines multiply when you are running on fumes. I have lived with a skull-crushing band of tension that has surrounded my temples for so long now, I am not sure I could even function without the pressure of feeling chronically irritated.

Itchy somewhere under the skin, between the muscle and bone, somewhere deep inside the tissue, which has been rubbed raw, prickly. Infected by an army of slow-moving insects whose miniscule mandibles rub together in delight as every inch of skin stings. The eyes twitch. The temples throb. The brain bleeds.

But after all, what's one more day, month, decade robbed of sleep and stuck squirming in a state of agitated limboessence, when you have an eternity of peace to eventually look forward to? That is if you are foolish enough to believe that yes!

death will be peaceful. It will caress like black velvet those shattered nerves and twisted muscles that have revolted now for so long that even beyond the grave they may still be screaming for relief.

A relief, like deep sleep, which I am convinced I may never, not in this lifetime or the next, ever experience.

2 POEMS
BOB HICOK

THE BUSY DAYS OF MY NIGHTS

Sometimes it's the zombie
or near-zombie movie, like the one from Monday night
in which in-bred mutant Appalachian cannibals
terrorized and tenderized six people in West Virginia
and it was obvious who'd be alive and pretty
at the end but not how the dead would become dead
and yummy. Then I leaned over my guitar
the color of dust and fingerprints, hours
of touching the same sounds and listening
with my stomach, I played softly
not to wake the sofa, with the whispers of my hands
while the thirty-nine windows of my life
took their black photos of the night. Next I walked
in the field behind our house, it's on a mountain,
everything's on a mountain here, grass
tall enough to look at eye to eye, grass
in a slight wind was a field of mothers
telling their babies to hush, I sat up high
where we think the sink-hole was and thought
of writers struggling with the in-bred
mutant Appalachian cannibal dialogue,
should it be uuuuugggh or mmmmmgh,
I found the Pleiades and remembered the lady-bug
walking across "At the Fishhouses," open on my desk,
a tiny orange pebble with six
upside-down canes for legs, it wobbled
over "Cold dark deep" as if considering and opened

its suitcase back and took out its top-secret wings,
flew seven inches above the ocean of the poem
and landed on "burn," and the gold sun
remembered me, came back a degree closer to winter
over the potato-shaped mountain and if I never
sleep again, I won't think of my eyes as bloodshot
so much as full.

2 A.M.

Frank in southside Grand Rapids stapled pages
of the Gideon to his stomach and stood
outside Social Services, he thought his soul
was in the streetlights—why they buzzed, flickered—
he was hit once by a truck and once
by a Cadillac with curb feelers
like everything gets touched.
By the time I got from my porch to Frank,
he was breathing like Toby getting high
with a paper bag over his mouth, ventilating
glue and I only talked to Frank twice, once
when he knocked on my door and asked
if I'd seen his face, once before the ambulance
drove him away from the blood he left in the shape
of Florida on the street.

I don't know why I miss things, I don't know what things
I miss, nostalgia comes with my body
because stars are running through me, carbon, loneliness,
all the elements, I am the remnant of light, of leaving.

Frank asked me to take care of his dog and looked
to his left, where there was an infinity of no dogs,
I said I would and have tried to care for something
that doesn't exist—me, you—tried to live
as if holy words are nailed to every gesture.

AWAKE!
And yes, I've been drinking, usually white
but I'm drinking red tonight, call it
Blood of Christ—brand wine, yet another reason
I'm not in advertising.
The city has a halo and the moon has a halo,
I'd like a halo, that's what my buzz is, a halo
around my brain, that must be
what Frank saw in the lights, a halo
like baby Jesus wore in paintings
below white winged angels, chubby babies
who knew better than to land on earth.

THE JEFFREY SPINDLER INTERVIEW: THE MAN WHO NEVER SLEEPS BY JEFFREY SPINDLER

MICHAEL KOENIG

Last month I had the distinct pleasure of interviewing Oscar Henderson, known to millions around the world as "The Man Who Never Sleeps." He'll be making several public appearances in the L.A. area next week.

Henderson, 39, rocketed to fame as the subject of his own reality-based television series, INSOMNIAC, on the USA Network. He spoke to me by phone last week from his home in El Cerrito, California.

Oscar, are you there?

Hi. Is this Jeff?

Jeffrey. It's great to finally talk with you.

Same here, man.

So, how does it feel to be awake all the time?

I'm tired, man. Really fucking tired.

You literally haven't been to sleep at all in the last ten years, is that right?

Yes, that's absolutely correct. I literally have not gotten a moment of sleep in all that time. I've got a certificate from my doctor to prove it. I can fax it to you, if you'd like.

AWAKE!

That won't be necessary.

In addition, a Qualified Medical Evaluator for the State of California has declared me to be 69% Permanently Disabled. This means that I get a check for $220 from the state every week. I think I'm horribly underpaid. After all, I'm a medical miracle, the only known case. The doctors were sure that I'd be dead by now.

Hey, man, tell me a little bit about yourself, okay? I like to find out something about the people who interview me. Otherwise this gets pretty fucking monotonous. You married?

Divorced.

Me, too. My wife left me when this whole sleepless thing started. You got any kids?

Two. A boy and a girl.

Sweet. I love kids.

So, back to your story for a minute. Is there anything the doctors can do for you?

For five years, I was under the care of Dr. Benton Pinkus, the pre-eminent sleep specialist in the State of California (or so he told me). My first appointment, I saw him for five minutes. He gave me tranquilizers. I just got groggy, as if someone had punched me in the head a few times.

I came back a few weeks later; told him it hadn't done any good at all. He gave me another prescription for sleeping pills, twice the dosage this time. I slurred my words, but did not fall asleep.

I started seeing him every week: Tuesdays at 4:30. We tried every conceivable therapy. He insisted that I stop using caffeine. I quit drinking coffee; my heart rate increased. He tried biofeedback. Nothing happened. They did a CAT scan; everything normal.

The eminent doctor found it simply unbelievable that I hadn't been to sleep at all. He put me in an auditorium and assigned shifts of medical students to watch me. They had me hooked up to machines that monitored my vital signs. What the fuck, I figured. My wife had left me; my life was no longer my own. I remained there for months, until somebody went to the newspapers. It was quite a scandal, in the Bay Area anyway.

And you still kept seeing Dr. Pinkus after that?

Well, it was covered by insurance. It would have been a hassle to change.

So what happened next?

It soon became obvious that my inability to get better was really starting to piss him off. The next time the nurse ushered me into his office, he looked crestfallen before I'd even opened my mouth.

"No luck?" he said.

I nodded.

He gave me a prescription for amphetamines that day. I wrote a novel, but every sentence was the same.

I didn't see Dr. Pinkus for six months after that. The appointment lasted five minutes. I swear he was drunk. He had this nagging cough, and he looked like he had put on fifteen pounds. I could see the tremors as he tried to shake my hand.

"You should see another doctor," Dr. Pinkus said. "All I know is that I can't cure you."

"You're the only doctor who's still willing to see me," I said.

"I'm not surprised," he said, wearing the most miserable smile that I had ever seen.

He told me to get drunk. It worked like caffeine for me. And as I was leaving the office, he followed me outside to smoke another cigarette.

Are you still under his care?

Dr. Pinkus died of a heart attack a year ago.

Do you feel somehow responsible for that?

No, not at all.

Have you tried alternative therapies?

Sure. I've seen acupuncturists, hypnotists and even a faith healer. Candles and incense were suggested. A pretty young woman insisted on playing the cello for me, topless, for hours at a time. I enjoyed the music a great deal (and enjoyed watching her play) but otherwise derived no benefit from it at all. Oh, and I once chanted for twenty-eight hours straight.

Did that do anything?

I lost my voice.

What's your average day like now? I assume you're seeing another doctor.

My current physician, Dr. Bernard Williams, insists that I stick to my normal sleep routine, as closely as I remember it anyway. Every night I wander through the house, turning out the lights and checking every door and window to make certain that they're securely closed. As soon as I finish brushing my teeth, I get into bed and turn out all the lights, having convinced myself that I'll be safe. But from the moment I close my eyes, my mind is a vaudeville of alarm.

At 8 a.m. I get out of bed and adjourn to the couch, where I sit and wait out the day. Any exposure to the sun leaves me feeling like I spent ten minutes in the microwave. It's like being an especially boring kind of vampire.

At least you probably get a lot more done than everyone else, with all that extra time that everyone else spends sleeping (laughs).

Nope. No more than I used to. I never realized how good I could get to be at wasting time until I started staying awake all day.

When did you first notice this condition? Was there some sudden event that happened, or was it gradual?

Well, I was cursed by a gypsy woman.

You were? Wow.

I cut her off in traffic. I'd never seen a woman curse like that.

That's pretty funny.

I always start out my speeches with that joke. It lightens the mood a little.

So what really happened?

You haven't heard this story? Okay, here goes. I used to work a night job, convenience store. It's a great job, if you enjoy conversing with drunks. You get so sick of those tinkling bells. Every time the door opens or closes, you hear them.

One night this guy came in, wearing a hooded sweatshirt. He hung around by the dairy case a long time. Fidgety. He came up to the counter and produced a loaf of bread and a gun.

"Give me all your money," he said. "NOW!"

I gave him the money I had in the cash register, told him the rest of it was in a safe, that I didn't have the key. White lie.

He took the wad of bills from my hand. I spotted a dollar bill on the floor and bent down to get it for him. I heard a gunshot, footsteps and then the tinkling bells. Was he gone? Could I be sure? I stayed down there. I'd thrown up on my shirt.

A few minutes later, I heard the bells again. I swore he was coming back to kill me.

"Hey," the voice said. "You open?"

I rose up from the floor and looked over the counter. A man was standing there with a six pack of beer. He grimaced as the vomit smell crept to him.

"I need cigarettes too. Winstons, unfiltered," he said.

"Leave it on the counter, okay?" I said.

"Just give me my smokes."

I went to get the cigarettes, which were locked up in a cabinet behind the counter. When I turned around, I noticed a bullet hole in the wall.

Jesus, that's scary.

It sure was. Anyway, as soon as the man left, I called the police. An officer came an hour later to take my statement, told me they'd get back to me if there was anything else they needed. I called my boss to let him know what had happened; he told me not to worry, they'd find someone else to fill in.

For the first couple of days, I didn't want to leave the house, even to get the mail, but I soon started feeling a lot better. I decided to celebrate by going to a late afternoon movie. Bargain matinee. I had a great time. Movies are a thousand times better when you're supposed to be working. I was feeling so good, I decided to walk home. Four guys jumped me from behind and hit me in the head with a plastic trash can. They took my wallet—with $37 in it.

I called the police non-emergency number, then called Judy at work. An officer came about forty-five minutes later, and I walked with him to the scene. The officer read me back my statement, and told me they'd be in touch with me if they needed anything further. He told me that a police photographer would be coming around, to document my injuries.

My wife got home at 7:30, bearing my favorite Chinese food. She asked me what happened; I told her the whole gruesome story. We turned on the TV and waited for the photographer. It wasn't until I turned around to pick up the remote that she noticed the blood. She offered me a warm washcloth. My head is evidence, I said. Don't bleed on the couch, she said.

Judy went to bed at 11. The photographer didn't arrive until after midnight.

"I guess I don't have to ask you what happened," he said, as soon as he entered our living room.

I didn't understand what he meant at first.

"You had a break-in?" he said.

"No," I said. "The place is just messy. I've been sick."

I have always done this—made up incredible excuses, even when there's really no need to. The embarrassment is too much for me—I panic.

The photographer took a few photos, then repeated what the officer had said—that they'd call me if they needed me. Of course, I never heard from them again.

Judy had offered to take me to the emergency room, but I decided against going to see a doctor. By then, I'd stopped bleeding, and it seemed better to try and sleep. I lay down on my pillow and waited, but every time I closed my eyes my mind would go crazy. I swore I heard voices, people planning to rob the place. It sounded like someone sawing at the lock, then the man outside said, "I'm the lookout. I'm waiting for my friends to get back."

I reached for my glasses on the night table and listened carefully for further proof, but all I could hear was the rain and the occasional car, skidding along the road. I tried turning over, but every time I did, Judy let out a gruesome sigh.

Eventually I went into the living room to calm my nerves, carrying my blankets over my shoulder, dragging them along the floor. I found my way to the chair that used to recline, and reached for the remote. The TV provided all the light I would need. I was looking for an old movie, something that did not demand much attention, but nothing caught my eye. I could hear Judy getting up to pee, so I came back to bed, but stayed awake until dawn. In the morning I could tell that she was mad at me, but couldn't bear to say. She knew that I was in pain, but hated being so tired.

I taped up plastic curtains over all the windows. The landlord from the building next door had just installed a security light, even though the place had been empty for three years. He's still trying to rent out the place, but he never returns anyone's calls. The light goes on at random intervals and shines directly into our bedroom. I've never been able to figure out what sets it off. Passing cars? Mice?

From then on, every night was the same. I'd try to sleep and fail, thoroughly waking Judy in the process. Eventually her compassion ran out. I knew this was torture for her. I encouraged her to find her own apartment; she promised to return when I found a cure. Our marriage had been merely serviceable before, but it might have lasted, who knows? Judy's gotten married again; we barely speak now. Obviously, there hasn't been anyone since. I'm so boring.

Now the black electrical tape is falling, and the curtains are covered in dust, but I still can't sleep. I've come to dread the thought of closing my eyes. It's a control issue, that's what my psychiatrist says. I'm not willing to submit to the blankness of sleep.

You must have been going through a really awful time emotionally.

Absolutely. I was trying to figure out why all this shit was happening to me all of a sudden. Over the next few weeks, I described the two incidents to all my friends. I became an expert at explaining my injuries in a fifty-word pitch. Judy would walk away in the middle of the conversation. Why did I have to belabor it? Even though I'd spent a month commiserating with her over an infected nail.

These conversations were ultimately unsatisfying since everyone that I talked

AWAKE!

with would either: a) chime in with their own experiences, which were inevitably far more horrible than mine or b) interrogate me, in order to determine my own degree of culpability.

"You shouldn't go out walking late at night."

It was seven in the evening.

"Isn't it a dangerous neighborhood?"

The cop who came out was surprised. He said that there aren't many muggings around here.

"Did you do anything to make them target you?"

No, I was just carrying my wallet in my pocket."

"Geez, I'm sorry."

Me too.

Now I have a lot fewer friends.

That's awful. But I still don't quite understand how that would cause you to go without sleep for ten years.

I was mugged two blocks from my house, man! I can see the exact spot where it happened from my porch. The convenience store where I worked is only a mile from here. The guys who did it, they probably live in my neighborhood. Fuck, man, they're probably watching me right now. I have to stay awake, to keep them at bay. I've got a gun, man. I'm holding it in my hand right now.

Why did you buy the gun?

Oh, you know. For peace of mind (laughs). I mean the worst thing is that they fucking got away with it, even if the cops eventually caught them for something else, because they've forgotten me and I remember them. Every motherfucking moment of my life the memory's there, lurking. I'll never be free again. Even if I blew them all away, there are still more of them out there. And silence is the worst, because I begin to listen closely. It amplifies my fear.

It gives you a heightened sense of reality?

Here's the crazy thing: ever since I stopped sleeping, all my dreams happen while I'm awake. Even now, I'm sitting here on the edge of my bed talking to you and I'm falling from a ten-story building.

Be careful!

My falling dream always ends the same way. I'm just about ready to hit the ground and then it rewinds back to the beginning. Immediately thereafter I'm walking around naked or taking a test I haven't studied for. I don't know, maybe I'm crazy. What do you think? You've been talking to me for a while. Do you think I'm crazy?

Here's how crazy I am: I'm walking down to the corner to buy a dozen eggs and I see the guys that mugged me, walking toward me, or maybe they aren't the guys, and I pull out a gun from my bag and shoot those fuckers down. The scene changes; the guys are gone. I look down and there's a gun in my hand and the barrel is still warm.

This happens to me every day. Every morning I read the newspaper from front to back just to make sure that I haven't committed some heinous crime. I watch nothing but news now, twenty-four hours a day, flipping around the dials for coverage of a major crime. CNN, MSNBC, Fox News, Court TV. Doesn't matter where it happened, it seems like next door to me. Someone is holding hostages in a school in Kentucky. There's a plot to blow up the Golden Gate Bridge. And the news anchors and reporters are fuckin' gleeful when the bodies hit the floor. It's their solemn duty to bring you all this carnage, LIVE! I don't really blame them, though. I'm not the only one watching.

There were fifty people murdered yesterday in the United States of America, and untold numbers of violent crimes, forcible rapes, robberies, assaults. Think about that shit and you're likely to blow your own head off. Or take someone else out first.

Jesus, we never saw anything like that on your TV show.

I tried, man. I was hoping to convey what it's like to live with this condition every day. But they cut all that stuff out. TV is always a compromise.

Nevertheless, a lot of us were surprised when the show was canceled after only one season.

AWAKE!

I'm fine with it, really. I'm on the college lecture circuit now, along with a couple of the kids from the *Real World*. And I've got a website, www.sleeplessguy.com. We sell autographed photos, nightlights, pajamas, you name it. Ten percent of the profits go to sleep-related charities! And there's a webcam 24/7 for sleeplessguy.com premium members. So, that's about it. You got all you need?

I think so. I'll call you, if anything comes up.

Say, where do you live, Jeff?

L.A..

Where in L.A.?

North Hollywood. Small place. I rent. Cost of living is scandalous here.

Maybe I could hang with you next week. Maybe stay over at your place. Give me your address. I'd love to meet your kids. You got custody?

Sure. I'll email it to you, how's that? Don't want to run up your cell phone bill.

Sounds great, man. You won't even know I'm there.

That seems like a great note to end this on. Thanks again for doing this.

No problem, man. My pleasure.

In Michael Koenig's dreams, Jeffrey Spindler is a freelance journalist who lives in Los Angeles.

IN THE SECULAR NIGHT
Margaret Atwood

In the secular night you wander around
alone in your house. It's two-thirty.
Everyone has deserted you,
or this is your story;
you remember it from being sixteen,
when the others were out somewhere, having a good time,
or so you suspected,
and you had to baby-sit.
You took a large scoop of vanilla ice-cream
and filled up the glass with grapejuice
and ginger ale, and put on Glenn Miller
with his big-band sound,
and lit a cigarette and blew the smoke up the chimney,
and cried for a while because you were not dancing,
and then danced, by yourself, your mouth circled with purple.
Now, forty years later, things have changed,
and it's baby lima beans.
It's necessary to reserve a secret vice.
This is what comes from forgetting to eat
at the stated mealtimes. You simmer them carefully,
drain, add cream and pepper,
and amble up and down the stairs,
scooping them up with your fingers right out of the bowl,
talking to yourself out loud.
You'd be surprised if you got an answer,
but that part will come later.
There is so much silence between the words,
you say. You say, The sensed absence

AWAKE!

of God and the sensed presence
amount to much the same thing,
only in reverse.
You say, I have too much white clothing.
You start to hum.
Several hundred years ago
this could have been mysticism
or heresy. It isn't now.
Outside there are sirens.
Someone's been run over.
The century grinds on.

THREE A.M.
MYLES GORDON

Lately I am
the astronomer after midnight

observing my household's
every move.

Three a.m. From my son's room
the rustle of covers

kicked off in sleep, whimpers growing
louder and more urgent.

Wrapped in
a bathrobe,

I go to him
before he's fully awake,

cradle his six-month body
against mine,

his balled fists wandering
until they come to rest

AWAKE!

beneath my chin. Night
by night I have already wiped

ten thousand tears
from his cheeks,

seen them glimmer
in the moonlight through the blinds,

felt their residue
on the back of my hand,

tasted their salt
with a brush of my lips,

each one a star
added to his personal constellation.

MONDAY

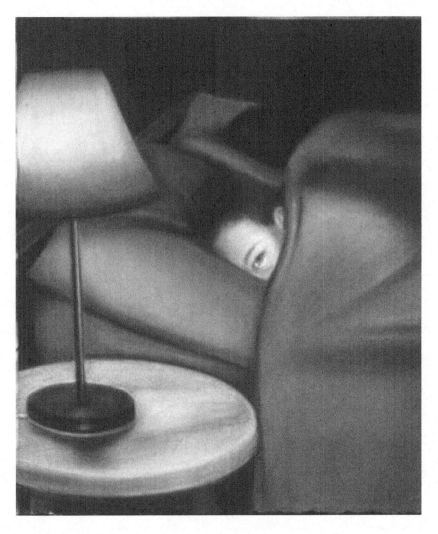

Nessun Dorma

SLEEP STUDY: EXAMINING MY LITTLE SLICES OF DEATH

Linda Werbner

How blessed are some people, whose lives have no
fears, no dreads, to whom sleep is a blessing that comes
nightly, and brings nothing but sweet dreams.

Bram Stoker, *Dracula*

Recently, the noose of debt was tighter than usual so I decided to loan out my body and my self-respect to science and market research groups. After all, I can tell a lie without blushing. Bottom line is there's not much I wouldn't do for a quick three hundred bucks.

It's no exaggeration to say that the driving principle in my life has been the quest to turn an easy buck. I trace my slothful instincts and aversion to so-called good, honest work to a book that I stumbled upon at the impressionable age of eighteen called *The Abolition of Work* when I was about to be catapulted into the vast electronic plantation of the modern workforce.

Bob Black's subversive masterpiece, with its imminently reasonable and logical argument that no one should ever have to work, was like drizzling kerosene over my bourgeois, programmed mind and then tossing in a match, and it spoiled my chances of ever holding a full-time job with a straight face and a sincere heart.

I've been a slacker ever since. And like most slackers, I also enjoy that condition that, to paraphrase Ambrose Bierce, only people of reason are blessed with: insomnia. Note—I didn't say *suffer* from because I don't see insomnia as an affliction. Sleep, those "little slices of death" that Edgar Allen Poe so loathed, usually doesn't find me until dawn. I drift through this world in a permanent, languid state of sleep deprivation. And I like it that way.

If you meet me, chances are good that I will yawn in your face at least once and

AWAKE!

if you don't burn, burn, burn like fabulous roman candles and if you're not exactly mad to live and mad to talk and NEVER say a commonplace thing à la Jack Kerouac, I could very well nod off like a junkie in your presence.

Happily, a fellow slacker turned me on to market research and focus groups and I've made some mind-bogglingly easy money as a participant in various studies. All I have to do is tell a few stretchers, embellish and lie through my teeth. When the market research folks needed someone who was planning to buy a new mattress (futons rule), owned a Gap credit card and shopped there (haven't, wouldn't and don't ever plan to) or drink light beer (that fizzy stuff ain't beer), I'm always ready to share my opinions. But there were no studies happening at the moment.

On to plan B. Monday morning found me scanning the medical research and clinical studies section of the newspaper for some relatively painless ways to get paid. The page was jumping with direct and indiscreet queries that would be inappropriate in polite company:

Are you menopausal?

Itchy, scaly skin?

Do you suffer from PMS?

Do you have mood swings?

Are you incontinent?

Are you shy? Do you have problems meeting new people?

Cocaine users and marijuana smokers needed!

Have you stopped taking hormone therapy?

Restless nighttime legs?

I zeroed in on the studies that didn't involve needles and overnight stays. I can barely stomach getting my blood pressure taken, let alone getting jabbed every hour for a blood sample. There was a promising depression study and one looking for healthy unmedicated right-handed individuals to talk about their memories of childhood. I nearly went with a dental study until I found out I couldn't brush my teeth for three weeks. Lightning struck when I saw the following:

DO YOU HAVE DIFFICULTY FALLING ASLEEP AT NIGHT?

Healthy volunteers needed for an insomnia research study.

No drugs—All treatments at home.

Qualified participants will receive $300.

Finally a chance to make some honest money. I was delighted at the thought of cashing in on my insomnia. This'll be a piece of cake. After a quick phone call to a breezy, upbeat lab assistant named Kenny, I came in that afternoon for a screening. I sat in a drab conference room of the sleep disorders clinic that smelt of bleach and microwave popcorn, waiting for Kenny to get off his cell phone. He was making a date to meet his girlfriend at a place called Wonder Bar.

Finally, on a cloud of Drakkar Noir, Kenny strolled in with a stack of papers. He looked like a sporty type in his sleek black tee-shirt made of some tight, shiny material, impeccably ironed chinos and expensive-looking sneakers. Outside it was below zero in Boston. I noticed that as we spoke, Kenny occasionally glanced at his bronzed biceps, as if checking to make sure they were still as magnificent as he remembered them.

"It is a non-invasive study but there are a few other things involved, including sleep diaries, electrodes for a three-day period, and a 24-hour urine sample, and halfway through the study you will receive a packet of exercises to use toward your sleep hygiene." Electrodes and urine samples didn't faze me. I just kept my eyes on the $300 prize.

"As part of the screening, I have to ask you some questions," said Kenny. "We have to screen out other illnesses."

"Fire away," I said, blithely.

"Do you snore?"

Someday I will.

"Do you stop breathing occasionally during sleep?"

Not that I'm conscious of.

"Do you sleepwalk?"

No, but I've always wanted to.

"Is there anything that you experienced or witnessed that has had a deep and disturbing impact on you?"

Yeah, that time dad drank a WD-40 cocktail when I was twelve. But the nice poison hotline lady told me what to give him and he was fine.

"Do you hear voices or see things that others can't?"

Who doesn't?

"Do you sometimes think that others are talking about or conspiring against you?"

Sure, but I don't let it bother me.

AWAKE!

Do you have periods of great happiness, excitability and anxiety followed by periods of sadness and depression?"

If I didn't then I wouldn't really be alive, you ding-dong.

"Do you think you have special powers that others lack?"

Of course I do, you shallow, walnut-brained, ugly bag of mostly water.

"No," I chanted with a composed, reassuring smile.

After he'd asked me all these questions, Kenny left to confer with the principal investigator, a charmless, brisk little man in a white turban with a cottony gray beard. A few minutes later, Kenny burst into the room and announced that I had passed the screening and I was officially in the study. I wanted to ask if I could get an advance on the $300 but I just gave a polite little smile.

The first three weeks of the study were a breeze. I filled in these sleep diaries detailing every nap I took, when I shut out the lights, how long it took to get to sleep, how many times I woke during the night, and what time I got out of bed. I'd never kept track of my sleep hygiene before but here it was in black and white. Count Dracula got more shut-eye than I. How am I able to function on so little sleep? When I mention how few hours of sleep I get to friends, they cluck their tongues and say, "I can't even function if I get less than 6 hours of sleep." A doctor friend told me that, for some people, prolonged sleep deprivation can result in a psychotic episode.

A month into the study I had a date with Kenny at the clinic to get "hooked up" as he called it. I was to wear a total of ten electrodes on my face, scalp and chest attached to an energy pack that I would wear around my waist. "Don't worry, they're small and there's some glue we use but it's water-soluble," he told me.

"Won't I look like the Bride of Frankenstein?" I asked, anxiously.

"Don't worry. It's not that bad," he said, snipping bits of gauze and half-watching the Friday Night Smackdown on the television suspended from the ceiling. At least it was dark outside and no one would see me, I thought.

Kenny began pouring an evil-smelling liquid all over my scalp that reminded me of Compound W. "Are you sure that won't melt my hair?" I asked with a grimace as he ground little disks into my head.

"Don't worry," Kenny said with a sigh, one eye cocked towards the television where the The Undertaker had Kurt Angle in a headlock.

Forty minutes later, I was hooked up and ready for the world. "The electrodes will record your heart rate and brain waves as you sleep," Kenny explained. "Just don't take a shower with these things on."

As I walked to the subway, my hood pulled snugly over my electrode-strewn face and head, it began to dawn on me how little we notice one another, how easy it is to be invisible. I ordered a coffee at Five Bucks and the barista didn't give me a second glance, the guy who rang up my toilet paper at the supermarket didn't seem the least bit curious about my electrodes, nor did the people on subway.

When I got home, my boyfriend was sitting on the couch watching *Star Trek*. He paused it and scrambled off the couch. "Let me see your electrodes!"

I grimly modeled the nest of colored wires streaming from my scalp and chin. "We should make love with those things on," he said, his eyes shining mischievously.

"Sorry, Max. But I'm not wired for that sort of thing. I can't even imagine how I'm going to sleep with all this shit on."

"You look like a cyborg," he observed. "Do you feel anything?"

"No, not really." We stood silently in the kitchen for a few moments. Then he said, "Hey, did you get funny looks when you walked down the street?"

"No, not at all."

He thought about this for a moment then his face broke into a grin. "I'd notice you if I saw you coming like that."

"I don't think so."

"No, I'd see you coming a mile away."

"No, probably not. I went into the drug store, the supermarket, Five Bucks and rode the subway, and I didn't get a single second glance."

"Did that make you feel sad?" he asked.

"No, it just made me think about how alienated we all are."

"Yeah, I guess," he said, absently. "Well, gotta get back to *Star Trek*. This is the one where Kirk and Spock have to fight to the death over a Vulcan maiden on Spock's planet." Max has seen this and every episode of *Star Trek* a hundred times and he can recite whole chunks of dialogue but he still likes to watch his favorites on Friday evenings. We used to watch them together and revel in the cheesy plots and bad acting. But we've both sort of drifted from that tradition.

I started sweeping, which I do when I am anxious or distracted. I enjoy cleaning. My broom found a collection of old popcorn kernels and some fossilized Meow Mix from our old cat Porkey, who died of kidney failure last summer. I also swept up an old photo that had fallen from the fridge door. It was a strip of three black and white photos Max and I'd taken at an old-fashioned photo booth at the Andy Warhol Museum in Pittsburgh. We were in town for an old friend's wedding—a big, fussy affair with rehearsal dinner, a commitment ceremony, and all kinds of weary pomp. In order to stave off the inevitable "So when are *you* guys gonna get married?" we lied and told everyone we'd finally tied the knot in a Justice of the Peace ceremony followed by a pot-luck reception in the driveway.

At one time, the refrigerator door was plastered with photos of us dressed in various costumes, dancing, mugging, kissing, and swinging from the chandelier. There was a photo of Max playing his accordion naked and one of me standing beside my late father dressed in identical oversized Mexican sombreros.

Where did all those pictures go, I wondered, staring at the naked white door. I sighed and stooped down to sweep the *shmutz* into the pan. I felt a tug and snag. Three of the electrodes that Kenny had so diligently glued on popped off and dangled stupidly from my energy pack. I took a kitchen magnet and posted the strip of photos in the center of the door and went into the living room to watch *Star Trek* with Max.

IT HURTS NOT TO FLY
Jonathan Messinger

The girl born with small wings on her back cannot conceive of flight, doesn't recognize the word. It is a cruel genetic joke. Like the ostrich and the penguin, she is in poor company.

The children at school say to her:

"If you hate it here so much, why don't you just fly away? No one would miss you."

To which she replies:

"I don't get it. What do you mean, 'fly'?"

It is unfair to call the wings on her back small, because she is small and they are in proportion to her body. She stands at 3-feet, 8-inches at twelve years of age. Her wings, always folded and chafing against her back, are a little shorter than a foot. Her eyes are pink and gossamer and beautiful. Her wings are black and red and of sandpaper.

She changes rooms for science class and moves slowly through the corridor. Today in science class her teacher is talking about aerodynamics. The teacher is a former army engineer and is a small man himself. He looks like a troll people sang about when people still sang about trolls. He is bald on his head and hairy on his hands. His name is Joe and his unpronounceable last name rhymes with his first, so everyone calls him Mr. Joe.

"If a missile is fired from a standing launch pad, there are several factors that must be accounted for. Does anyone know what they are?" The class is accustomed to Mr. Joe's army examples and lets him continue on his own. "Well, first there's the angle of the launcher. Then there's the weight of the missile and gravitational pull. Then, there's the, get this, *curve of the Earth*. Pretty neat, huh?" Mr. Joe has drawn sweeping lines and small objects on the blackboard. The objects look to the girl born with small wings on her back like tiny bars of soap.

"But there's one thing we haven't accounted for here, and it's very important. Can anyone tell me what it is?" There's a silence like between songs on a record. "How about you, you can tell me what I've forgotten." He looks directly at the girl born with small wings on her back. "What does every bird or plane or baseball have to worry about in flight?"

"Can a baseball worry?" asks the girl.

"You know what I mean," says Mr. Joe, wincing at his grinding jaw.

"I don't know that last word you said," says the girl. She looks down to write its possible spellings: flite, flyte.

Mr. Joe is angry. He doesn't appreciate snide remarks. In the army, he learned that dealing early with this sort of dissent was important. An emotional cautery. He picks up a blackboard eraser to hurl at her. His brain whispers to his arm that this is not the right course of action, but his instincts have been trained to think like our nation's army and so it summons our country's unspoken military motto: *We've done it before and gotten away with it. Why stop now?*

The eraser knuckles through the air like a clumsy sea creature. The children sitting in the rows before the girl born with small wings on her back have no trouble getting out of the way. The girl looks up to see the eraser but doesn't understand what she is seeing. The eraser, colliding with the girl's head, releases a cloud of yellow chalk particles. It's a kind of bomb, the kind that makes schoolchildren laugh. As destructive as any.

"Now do you understand that last word?" says Mr. Joe.

The girl, embarrassed by the laughter and surprised to find herself covered in an almost radioactive yellow dust, sinks in her chair.

"Do you understand that the eraser flew?" asks Mr. Joe.

The girl thinks, "Flew: F-l-o-o."

She looks at Mr. Joe, and because she seems to disappoint adults so easily, wants to please him. She says, "Is floo like dropping?"

At home, her mother asks again about her sleep. Since her father left, the girl born with small wings on her back sleeps in fits, and it seems to her mother as though she has not slept in several days. The girl does not argue. There is a guilt to her mother's tone, and she gives her daughter a toy as a diversion; a beginner's collector set of military planes. The girl doesn't open the packaging because she doesn't like to destroy things and to her the packaging is as much a thing as what it holds inside. It is plastic bubbles on cardboard. There are tiny brown, green and gray objects inside the bubbles that look like vicious little bugs. With the bugs is a translucent blue plastic suitcase.

The girl born with small wings on her back tries to remember where she has seen these things before. She remembers now how her father used to make things from paper, things that looked like these little things, only white and large. Back when her father was still here, hadn't moved away. Back when her father still made things.

The girl born with small wings on her back lies on her stomach, the sheets of her bed cold against her bare skin. She can't sleep. Her mother thinks it's because of the pain in her back, but really it's her dreams. In the dreams she walks the streets of a thriving city among strangers who grab her by the hand and pull her along as if her feet were wheels. She is passed around for some time until, at the edge of the city, she falls into a gray sky. Her nightmare is to fall and fall and she is powerless to stop it and so she never does. When she finally wakes, she thinks there is no solution to prevent her falling except to stay awake. Still, these nightmares cling to her for days; wispy daydreams that by the third day feel like clinging hallucinations.

As she lies there, her mother lifts the wings gently from the girl's back and salves her skin with a Chinese lotion made of insect blood and rare herbs, a nightly ritual to try lull the girl. Beneath the wings, the girl's skin is a horrifying topography of scars and bruises and scabs that never heal. Her sandpaper wings are like machines against her delicate skin. She never thinks to lift them.

She stares down at the gift from her mother and reads the words over and over again, "Keep your tiny planes in a suitcase!"

"Mom, what are planes?" she asks, not looking back.

"They're what fly people to different places." Her mother checks herself, knowing the word "fly" will only confuse her daughter. "It's how we travel."

"So flying is traveling," says the girl born with small wings on her back. Why had no one told her? She will simply fly to see her father.

"You should sleep, honey," says her mother, the bed rising as she stands.

The girl born with small wings on her back nods, but she knows she won't. For the first time, she is energized by her insomnia.

At school, the children are abuzz. The girl born with small wings on her back announced at recess that she plans to fly for the first time that day. For the children, it is like they have finally elected a president they wanted after years of an oppressive regime. They party at recess the way children party, by running in circles and climbing on each other and falling from playground equipment until at least half of them are hurt and crying. When they line up to go back inside, their faces streaked and blotched with red, their energy has been spent. The girl born with small wings on her back doesn't know what the big deal is. She only wants to fly. To travel.

In class Mr. Joe can't help tittering around the girl. He's heard the news and is curious like a child. Also, he feels guilty about his behavior the day before, even though, still thinking like the Army, he blames the girl for his aggression.

AWAKE!

"You're going to be something," he says to the girl as he walks by her desk. The girl born with small wings on her back thinks Mr. Joe has lost his mind. She pretends not to notice how sleepy she grows.

After school, she runs home and takes her mother's old suitcase from under the eaves. She packs it with her pillow, two blankets, her salve, a shirt and a pair of pants. Still in the packaging, she slides her tiny planes and their toy suitcase into her mother's luggage. She closes it and there is so much room in the bag that the girl born with small wings on her back thinks maybe the bag could float in the air, a type of dropping. Her wings itch her back.

She takes a free shuttle that stops at the train platform near her home and is patient as the driver makes the rounds. Confused to see such a young girl by herself, the driver strikes up a conversation.

"Where ya headed?" he asks.

"To see my father," she replies. The coach's cushions seem to drag her toward sleep.

"Where does he live?"

"I am flying to see him," is all she says, confident that is all that's needed. The word *fly* is heavy to her now. She knows what everyone has been asking.

At the airport, she immediately makes her way to the bathroom. She enters an empty stall and stands on the toilet, removes her shirt. She is yellowed from not sleeping but under the fluorescent light looks white. She spreads her wings for the first time in a long time, and the effect is like a waterfall of adrenaline, like an amputee growing a new limb.

She spreads them magnificently, shakes them and the bathroom smells of animal. Still, she drops them again against her back. Puts her shirt back on. Goes out onto the concourse. She approaches the security check and, while the guard is busy inspecting someone's shoes, opens the suitcase. She crawls into the suitcase, seals it shut with a tiny piece of cloth she's tied to the zipper. She wraps herself in the blanket and lays her head against the pillow. Her back aches, but the spreading of her wings has released endorphins that make her euphoric. She begins to drift off to sleep, as a lullaby repeats the sentence on her lips.

"I am flying to see my father."

"I am flying . . ."

From "The Mezzanine"
Nicholson Baker

Although earplugs are essential for getting to sleep, they are useless later on, when you are awakened with night anxieties, and your brain is steeping in a bad fluorescent juice. I slept beautifully through college, but the new job brought regular insomnia, and with it a long period of trial and error, until I hit on the images that most consistently lured me back to sleep. I began with Monday Night at the Movies title sequences: a noun like "MEMORANDUM" or "CALAMARI" in huge three-dimensional curving letters, outlines with chrome edgework of lines and blinking stars, rotating on two axes. I meant myself to be asleep by the time I passed through the expanding O, or the dormer window of the A. This did not work for long. In the belief that images with more substance to them, and less abstract pattern, would encourage the dreaming state, I pictured myself driving in a low fast car, taking off from an aircraft carrier in a low fast plane, or twisting water from a towel in a flooded basement. The plane worked best, but it didn't work well. And then, surprised that I had taken so long to think of it, I remembered the convention of counting sheep. In Disney cartoons a little scene of sheep springing lightly over a stile or a picket fence appears in a thought-cloud above the man in the bed, while on the soundtrack violins accompany a soft voice out of 78 records saying, "One, two, three, four . . ." I thought of story conferences in Disney studios back in the golden days of cartoons: the look of benign concentration on the crouching animator's face as he carefully colored in the outline of a suspended stylized sheep one frame farther along in its arc, warm light from his clamp-on drafting-table lamp shining over the pushpins and masking tape and the special acetate pencil in his hand—I was soon successfully asleep. But though this Disney vision achieved its purpose, it felt unsatisfactory: I was imagining sheep, true, but the convention, which I wanted to uphold, called for counting them. Yet I didn't feel that there was any point to counting what was obviously the same set of animated frames recycled over and over. I needed to pierce through the cartoon and create a procession of truly differentiable sheep for myself. So I homed in on each one in its approach to the hurdle and looked for the individuating features—some thistle prominently caught, or a bit of dried mud on a shank. Sometimes I strapped a number on the next one to jump and gave him a Kentucky Derby name: Brunch Commander, Nosferatu, I Before E, Wee Willie Winkie. And I made him take the jump very slowly, so that I could study every phase of it—the crumbs of airborne dirt floating slowly toward the lens, the soft-lipped grimace, the ripple moving through the wool on landing. If I wasn't off by then, I backed up and reconstructed the sheep's entire day; for I found that it was the *approach* to the jump, rather than the jump itself, that was sleep-inducing. Some sheep had probably reported for work around noon several towns over, tousled and fractious. Around two in the afternoon, while at my office, expecting a rough night, I had (I imagined) placed a call to one of the shepherd-dispatchers: Could she send out some random number of sheep not greater than thirty to arrive outside my apartment by 3:30 a.m., for counting? The practiced crook of the sheep dispatcher travels over her herd, pointing: "You, you, you"; she repeats my address again and again to her nodding subjects; and my personal flock departs fifteen minutes later, with a voucher to be signed on arrival. All that afternoon they cross village greens, wade brooks, and trot along the median valleys of highways. While I am eating dinner with L., they are still miles away, but by bedtime, 11:30 p.m., I can spot them with my binoculars coming over a rise: tiny bobbing shapes next to a foreshortened Red Roof Inn sign, still in the next county. And at 3:30 a.m., when I need them badly, they bustle up, exhilarated from their journey: I put aside the unwritten thank-you letter I have been writhing over, log the sheep in and pay them off, and the first few begin lofting themselves over the planks and milk crates I have assembled out front, their small pink tongues visible with the effort, the whites of their sheep eyes showing; one, two, three . . . and then I have become a very successful director of fabric-softener commercials—the agency needs lush shots of jumping sheep; their fleece has to read as golden in the failing sunlight, and the greens of the countryside have to be inconceivably full-throated. I shampoo each sheep myself; I comfort the weepers; I read to the assembled flock from Cardinal Newman's *Idea of a University* to heighten their sense of purpose and grace, and I demonstrate to them how I need them to *send* their plump torsos airborne, hike *up* their rear legs for an added boost, *throw* their heads back for drama, and always, always lead in their landing with the forehoof. I have them cue through a rolled-up script: "Okay, number four. Lighter footfalls. Now thrust. Up. And the rear legs! More teeth! Show strain! Now some nostril! And over!" Lately I have found that the last thing in my mind before resumed unconsciousness is often the dwindling sight of one lone sheep, who, having cleared my hurdle and been checked off, full of relief and the glow of accomplishment, is hurrying over farther hills to his next assignment, which is to leap an herbal border in slow motion for L., awake with worries of her own beside me.

INSOMNIA™
CATIE LAZARUS

INSOMNIA (IN*SOM*NIA): Latin for "in slumber not me." Noun (not proper or improper). Pronunciation: in-'säm-nE-ya. According to Webster's Dictionary insomnia is a prolonged and usually abnormal inability to obtain adequate sleep, also referred to as agrypnia, albeit only by an anal-retentive, know-it-all show-off, a.k.a Webster's. Insomnia is characterized by a "difficulty with sleeping" presumably not while pushing paper around in your windowless cubicle.

Insomniacs can experience sleep problems for different periods of time, falling into three overall categories: transient, short-term, or chronic. Chronic means every night, most nights, or several nights each month, but never many or few nights, at least rarely. Physicians indicate that sleeplessness may also be caused by bad sleep habits, which include underwater sleeping, falling asleep at the wheel, be it a golf cart or school bus, and/or sleeping while vomiting.

SIDE EFFECTS OF INSOMNIA:

1.) Lack of sleep can lead to difficulty feeling a "spring in your step," "seizing the day," and "seeing the present as a gift." One antidote is to spam block the annoying relative who forwards emails like a pseudo-religious ode about a Pakistani refugee who almost died during a moose flu epidemic but learned to love again, and so can you, by forwarding this email to thirty-seven others.

2.) Not being able to sleep (and not because Rachel Weisz is begging to go down on you) may leave you feeling super-, hyper-, uber-, or ultra-stressed about how you are going to function. Remind yourself of how little you do know, be it about credit card identity theft, nuclear arms, or the plight of the Druze, and yet you still "function."

3.) Sometimes an inability to sleep can lead to fantasies of grandeur.

Warning signs include being interviewed by Barbara Walters as her last great catch, practicing your Oscar, Nobel Prize, or "I quit, boss" speech, and trusting a political leader.

4.) Agrypnia (see above) may result in a loss of appetite, which may, in turn, result in weight loss. Use caution when exercising insomnia as an appetite suppressant, although less caution than if you suffer from Dengue. Physicians recommend an alternative of exercising more and eating less, like masochistic, traditional Japanese women.

5.) More likely if you are milling around the house at odd hours, regardless of your cable package, your appetite but not your metabolism may increase. Late night snacking can lead to bingeing which could lead to a book deal, for your story, "The Nighttime Nosher," "Sleepless Stuffer," or "Fatso: A Love Story."

6.) Without adequate sleep you may appear sallow, pasty, or otherwise thin-skinned. Minor irritations include: eye circles, puffy, bloodshot eyes, black and blue bruising, or puss oozing from your retina. If any two of these signs (but not three) are accompanied by a spinal cord injury, you may or may not have a spinal cord injury.

RESEARCH:

Medical professionals define insomnia as a minor mental health disorder, and the symptoms may be viewed as "challenges" or "opportunities for growth." Perhaps you will not suffer as much as an orphaned Eritrean bastard who lives with typhoid, HIV, and a club foot, but you will struggle more than a trophy wife, no matter how often she must oblige her husband/account manager and how unattractive he is.

According to a study conducted by the leading anesthetic sleep medication, Snoremore (Generic label) in conjunction with Dr. Harrison Hyman, a dermatologist, "sleeping helps." Dr. Hyman was paid a seven-digit salary for this finding based on a qualitative, pseudo-scientific study of a sample pool of seven subjects, one of whom may or may not have had mononucleosis, pink eye and/or athlete's foot. The intern doing the actual work for Dr. Hyman found that insomniacs generally (at least two or more subjects but no more than three) face at least two but no more than one of the following criteria:

1.) Trouble falling asleep, even if your hotel offers free porn that your spouse will never know about.

2.) Difficulty staying asleep (also known as ruminating about an attorney charging you for a brief email exchange).

3.) Waking up too early, which for 107.3% of the population who don't have trust funds is a daily dilemma.

4.) Lack of interest in sex with your partner, which is often confused with a lack of interest in sex.

5.) Trouble trusting your president; knowing that if you murdered him you are stuck with the vice-president; recognizing that the other party has no real viable leaders and you and your family are screwed not just for the next four years, but forever.

6.) Not feeling rested when you wake up, i.e., anyone with a boundary-less mother-in-law who is three hours ahead but calls to share her recurring dream about you cleaning out the attic, when the only dream worth sharing before noon is Martin Luther King, Jr's.

7.) Desire to write a blog, record a podcast or short film about not sleeping, which will only add to the mind-numbing amount of self-indulgent blather available. Stay away from sending snarky emails to your boss about her corrosive management style, your ex about cheating on him, or your best friend about her lopsided nose job.

Preventive Measures:

If and when you first start taking any sleep medication, use extreme care while doing anything that requires complete alertness, such as cooking, managing a staff, and staying married.

The most common side effects of sleep medicine include:

Trouble sleeping, dizziness, toe pus, lightheadedness, daytime drowsiness, swelling of the right calf, diarrhea, tremors, speaking in tongues, difficulty with coordination, lockjaw, drooling, small pox, and paranoia. Follow your doctor's instructions about how to take medication and if you experience any unusual, erratic, or dangerous behavior be mindful when operating firearms and explosives, such as hand grenades.

Active Ingredients:

Lethal, addictive elements not yet legal in Peru, Canada and Guam. Consult your doctor if you are breast-feeding, have ever inhaled or use water with fluoride, a.k.a tap water.

Non-active Ingredients:

Water, lemon zest, two ounces of paprika mixed with cumin and six organic shallots, and ink.

Subject Pool:

Drop-in self-selected pool of non-English speakers who filled out surveys for five hours in the middle of the workday for no money.

Other Non-Fatal Treatments:

1) Engage in sex with or without your partner, but not with mine.

2) Write a bestselling novel.

3) Create the final Middle East peace treaty.

4) Learn Finnish.

5) Sell your roommate's or partner's belongings on e-Bay.

Do not substitute this helpful pamphlet with medical advice from your primary care physician who knows your individual case history from the four minutes he spends with you annually. To purchase products, including wristbands, tongue depressors, and other must haves from our online store, please have a credit card available and log onto www.snowme.com.

FROM THE INSOMNIA DRAWINGS
Louise Bourgeois

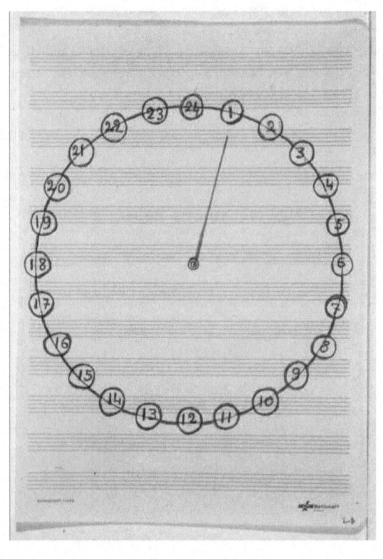

The Insomnia Drawings (detail), 1994-1995
220 mixed media works on paper of varying dimensions
Daros Collection, courtesy Cheim & Read, New York
Photo: Christopher Burke

INSOMNIA
BETH WOODCOME

I know a sadness has been building
from the distance of a Scandinavian country.
We stood on the pier and helped the dog
over the darkness of a brackish sea and into the boat.
It was only a foot or so of risk, wasn't it?
Or did it feel much further when she seized in your hands?

There is only one person to think of when you lose that person.
It so happens that every night is where you want them back.
I feel like I am that dog: restive, wakeful, undocked.
Now. This is my night, my bed, and I'm the animal in it.

TRAVELS WITH PAUL
ARTHUR BRADFORD

I had been fired from my job for a stupid indiscretion and needed to leave town. I packed up my belongings quickly and caught a ride with an acquaintance who was headed out west. There was no good reason for going west except that it was someplace new and this acquaintance had offered me a ride. I say "acquaintance" because I'd only met him once before. He was an Irish fellow named Paul O'Malley and he was the cousin of a woman I used to date, or maybe they were lovers, I don't know. She had introduced him to me one night in a bar by saying, "This is my cousin Paul."

Paul was passing through town on his way west and announced that he would be gone in the morning. I saw him two weeks later though, right after I'd been fired from that job. He was still in town, looking a little dazed and strung out.

"I haven't slept in three days," he told me.

"I thought you were going west," I said.

"I am."

"But you said you were leaving two weeks ago."

"I got hung up. Wait, two weeks? It hasn't been that long."

"Yes it has."

"Oh." Paul scratched his head. He hair was thinning at the top. He was a skinny guy with a long neck and an enormous Adam's apple which bobbed up and down when he spoke. He needed a shave too, or maybe he was growing a beard. The stubble was at that awkward scruffy halfway point.

"I got fired from my job," I told Paul. "I'd like to leave town."

"You want to ride with me? I'll leave tomorrow."

This idea seemed to perk Paul up. He clapped his hands together and rubbed his fuzzy chin.

"Sure, yeah, okay," I said.

"We'll leave in the morning."

"Great, fine."

We left two days later. Paul picked me up at my place, still looking tired and run down.

"I can't sleep," he said. "I can't even shut my eyes."

"What's wrong with you?" I asked him.

"Nothing. Insomnia. I'm fine."

"You don't look fine."

"Well I feel fine," he said, "I just can't sleep."

"Listen," I told him, "I don't want any funny business. I just need a ride out of town."

"Sure, right, I understand that," he said.

Paul's car was a small Ford hatchback. It was already crammed full with his stuff so I had to leave several of my belongings behind. I left them with a friend with the understanding that I'd return for them later. I never did. Anyway, we hit the road and began to head west. Paul's car was equipped with a set of very worn out seats. The one I was sitting in, the passenger seat, had something wrong with the backrest. If I leaned back it would slope off to one side and I'd twist around uncomfortably. I'd been hoping to get a little sleep while he drove, but I could see now that this wouldn't be possible.

After about three hours of driving Paul pulled off the highway and stopped in front of a pizza shop. He unbuckled his pants and pulled them down to his knees. Then he looked at me.

"What are you doing?" I asked him.

"I thought maybe you'd like to give me a blowjob," he said.

"No," I said. "No, I wouldn't."

Paul pursed his lips and nodded his head.

"Alright," he said, pulling up his pants in a hurry. He put the car in gear and sped back out onto the highway.

Now things were awkward between us. We drove for a few hours in silence. A heavy rain began to fall as we crossed the state line into Ohio. When the big trucks passed by, water splashed against our windshield and threatened to push the little car right off the road. Paul had to jerk the steering wheel this way and that to keep us on course.

"Are you getting tired?" I asked Paul. "I can drive. I'm a good driver."

"That's okay," said Paul. "I like to drive."

But then a few minutes later he said, "Actually, I'm getting sick of this. Maybe you should drive."

"Okay," I said.

He pulled over and we switched seats, running around the car quickly so as to not get too wet from the rain.

The driver's seat was even less comfortable than the passenger seat. I felt like I was sitting in a bucket. The little hatchback was difficult to operate as well. The clutch was loose and I was never quite sure when it would kick into gear. Out on the highway the big trucks cruised by and pushed us around like a rowboat on a stormy sea.

"I hope this rain stops soon," I told Paul.

"Oh, it will," he said.

Paul leaned back and tried to shut his eyes. Every time he did though he could only keep them closed for a few seconds. Then he'd pop them open and his head would snap forward.

"What was that?" he'd ask me.

"Nothing," I'd say, "I'm just driving."

"I can't even take a nap," said Paul, finally. "This is a big pain in the ass."

"Maybe you should take some sleeping pills," I suggested.

"Oh, I won't do that," said Paul. "That's a vicious cycle. Everyone knows that."

"Okay," I said.

A while later Paul sat up and said, "Are you trying to kill me?"

"No," I said, "I'm not. I was trying to help."

Paul stared at me with his bloodshot eyes and I could see then that if he didn't get some sleep soon things were seriously going to unravel.

"I'm going to pull over," I told Paul. "Maybe I should get out."

"What do you mean?" he asked.

"I think I should get out here," I said. "I've gone far enough."

"What are you talking about?" said Paul. He rubbed his face and leaned forward in his seat. "You said you wanted to come west. We're only in Ohio."

"I know that," I told him. "I just think you need some sleep. We both do, actually."

"Well, that's fine, but don't abandon me here. We've got a long ways to go. I'm not doing this alone."

"You were going to do it alone before," I pointed out.

"Oh don't pull that on me now," said Paul. He slapped his hand against the window. The rain was letting up, at least. I thought Paul was going to cry. We passed by a sign for Zanesville and Paul said, "Hey!"

"What?"

"I know someone in Zanesville."

"We passed it already."

"No, let's stop there. She's a nice gal. She'll give us food. I haven't seen her in years. She'll be happy to see me."

I wasn't so sure about that, but I though this might be my chance to make a clean break, so I pulled off at the next exit and we backtracked to Zanesville. It was a muddy town situated on the bank of a river. Paul had me drive around in circles for over an hour looking for a street name with the word "Cherry" in it.

"Cherryvale. Cherryville, something like that."

When we found the street it was called Vine Street.

"Cherries grow on vines," explained Paul. "They're vegetables. They grow on vines."

After some more aimless driving along this street we eventually stopped in front of a brown cottage with a mailbox shaped like a football.

"This is Alberta's house," said Paul. "This is it!"

"Are you sure? How do you know?"

"I was here before," he said, "I spent a week and a half here. I remember this place."

We walked up to the front door and Paul pounded upon it.

"We go way back," Paul said to me. "We had a good thing going, me and Alberta."

"When was this?" I asked.

"Six years ago," said Paul. "Or maybe seven. She'll remember me."

He knocked on the door again but it appeared that no one was home. Paul leaned over a hedge and looked through the window.

"Hmmm," he said. He tried turning the door handle but it was locked. He looked back in the window again.

"We shouldn't go in there," I said to him.

"I know, I know."

We sat down on the doorstep and watched the cars drive by. I had seen a bus station back in town when we were driving around. I thought maybe I could catch a ride over there and find a bus headed west.

"I think I'll head over to the bus station," I said to Paul.

"Oh no," he said. "Oh no you don't. You haven't even met Alberta."

"She's not home," I pointed out. "She might not come back for days."

Paul thought about this for a moment. "She wouldn't do that," he said. "She wouldn't just disappear."

"You haven't seen her for six years," I said. "You have no idea what she might be up to."

"Look," Paul said, "do you trust me or not?"

I could have told him honestly then that I did not. What kind of question was that? But instead I said, "I trust you, Paul."

We sat on the step for a while longer. Paul shut his eyes and rested his greasy head on my shoulder. I was afraid to move because I knew he needed sleep and I didn't want to wake him up. We sat like that for perhaps twenty uncomfortable minutes and then a pick-up truck rumbled to a stop in front of the house. Two teenagers, a boy and a girl, both overweight and pale, got out and began walking cautiously towards us, holding hands. I jiggled my shoulder and Paul opened his eyes.

"That's not Alberta," he said to me. He shut his eyes again.

"They're walking this way," I told him.

"So what?" said Paul. He refused to move.

The pudgy girl squinted at us and said something into her boyfriend's ear. They stopped walking and looked us over. The girl was wearing a lot of dark make-up around her eyes. She had dark lipstick on too. The boy had stringy black hair and was wearing a hefty pair of black boots with many buckles. The two of them could have been dressed up for Halloween, but it wasn't that time of year.

It appeared that no one else was going to do any talking so I said, "Hello."

"Hi," said the girl.

Paul still had his head resting on my shoulder and I jerked it off so that he would sit up. He rubbed his eyes and blinked at the rotund young couple in front of us.

"What the fuck happened to you two?" he said.

"I live here," said the girl.

"Here?" said Paul.

"Yes."

Paul stood up and turned around as if he didn't know there was a house behind him. I stood up too, trying to look apologetic.

"This is Alberta's house," Paul said.

"Right," said the girl. "She's my mother."

Paul eyed her skeptically. "Your mother? What's your name?"

"Linda," said the girl.

"Linda!" Paul cracked a smile and moved towards her. The girl stepped back, away from him. The boy shuffled uneasily in his enormous boots.

"I know your mother," Paul said to the girl. "And I know you too. I remember when you were just a little whippersnapper wetting your pants every morning. You and me used to read the comics in the paper together. Boy, you've really grown up. Gotten fat, actually. It's me, Paul O'Malley, remember? What the fuck are you two doing to your faces anyway?"

Linda said, "I don't remember you."

"Sure you do," said Paul. "Seriously, what is that in your lip, a fish hook?" He was referring to a ring which Linda had stuck through a piercing in her lip. The boy had one too, except it was stuck through his eyebrow.

"My mom's not home yet," said the girl. "She's at work. She gets home at eight."

"Great, no problem," said Paul. "We'll wait inside."

He stepped aside so that Linda could get by. Linda and the boyfriend walked past us and opened the door.

"Don't do anything stupid," said Linda. "My mom's boyfriend will kick your ass if you mess anything up."

"It's cool," said Paul, "I just want to take a nap."

The house was cluttered with various knick-knacks, a lot of stuffed animals and products associated with the Cleveland Browns football team. We sat in the living room and talked to the kids for a while. Linda's boyfriend was named Ryan. They went to school together and had been dating for about three months. Ryan pulled out a pipe and offered us some marijuana but Paul wouldn't touch it. He said it would keep him awake.

Linda and her boyfriend got bored with us and went into her bedroom and shut the door. Paul poured himself a glass of milk from the refrigerator, sat back down on the living room couch, and turned on the television.

"I'm going to leave now," I said.

"No fucking way," said Paul.

"Yes, I'm leaving."

"Just stay here until I fall asleep," he said. "I haven't slept in five days."

AWAKE!

"Turn off the TV then. Go to sleep."

Paul turned off the TV, drank his milk, and lay back on the couch. I was tired too and decided I could use a little rest. I lay down on the shag carpeted floor and shut my eyes. Paul kept shifting about on the couch and cursing so I found it hard to actually sleep. I kept thinking I heard Alberta coming and I would sit up, afraid she'd find us lying there and confusion would ensue.

A rhythmic thumping noise drifted out of Linda's bedroom and Paul said, "Hey, those kids are humping in there."

He jumped up and before I could stop him he was knocking on Linda's door saying, "Stop that, you fat little rabbits!"

He burst through the door and indeed the two of them were naked rolling about amongst the stuffed animals on her single bed.

Linda said, "Will you shut the door?"

Paul said, "Not until you get dressed!"

It was an uneasy standoff, but eventually Paul left them alone and lay back down on the couch. There was no more noise from Linda's room and I finally fell asleep on that shag carpet floor. When I woke up Paul was in the kitchen coughing and making a big racket. I went in there and he was kneeling on the floor with his head stuck in the oven. The room smelled like gas.

"What's going on here?" I asked.

"Fuck," said Paul. "Shit."

He was trying to inhale the gas fumes and kill himself but he couldn't create a proper seal around his head so the gas was escaping into the room. I grabbed his legs and pulled him away from the oven.

"Leave me alone!" he cried out.

We wrestled about on the kitchen floor and during the struggle Paul tried to kiss me, his hairy face and puckered lips lunging towards me.

"I'm not a gay," he said. "I can't sleep. Just kiss me."

Finally I got him to calm down and we sat together on the linoleum floor breathing heavily, sucking in that gas-filled air.

"I've got a headache," said Paul.

There was a clicking sound from Linda's room and then a warm blue flame rushed across the hallway floor and burst into the kitchen with a loud hot boom. For a brief second the whole room filled up with a wall of fire and then suddenly we were sitting in the charred kitchen with little flames flickering around us. The paper towels were burning and so were some potholders and the curtains. Paul and I stood up and slapped at the flames and threw water everywhere. Ryan came in and helped us. We yanked the curtains down and tossed them in the sink. A smoke alarm went off and its shrill noise drove us nuts until Paul swatted it down with a broom. After a while we managed to put out all the fires in the house. The shag carpet was seared black and some of the stuffed animals were still smoking. Linda was crying in her bedroom. The place smelled awful now, like burnt plastic. Paul and I noticed that our hair was singed too. Our eyebrows were mostly gone and the skin on our faces was red and burned.

"We could have died," said Paul.

"That's what you were trying to do," I reminded him. "You had your head in the oven."

Ryan apologized because it was his lighter which had set off the flame.

"That's what you get for smoking those doobies, you little fornicator," said Paul.

"I'm sorry," said Ryan. He was really shaken up. We all were.

It was nearly eight o'clock and Alberta would soon be coming home. Paul decided maybe she wouldn't be so happy to see him after all. He and I had a brief discussion away from the kids and then we dashed out to his little hatchback and drove away, leaving Linda and Ryan to explain the mess we'd left behind.

"That Linda has really changed," said Paul. "I remember when she was just a cute little cartoon watcher. Now look at her, all plumped up and punched full of metal."

A police car passed us going the other way, its lights flashing and siren blaring. Paul began to get paranoid and insisted that we ditch the car. That was fine with me.

We parked the car on a side street and walked over to the bus station where we purchased two tickets to Seattle, a thirty-seven hour ride. As we waited for the bus to show up Paul lay down across three of those plastic bus stop seats and he finally fell asleep. It was chilly in there and those seats looked about as comfortable as a pile of rocks, but there he was, snoring away. I briefly considered waking him up when the bus arrived and it was time for us to load on, but then I thought better of it. He was still sleeping like a baby, curled up contentedly under those pale flourescent lights, when we pulled away and headed west without him.

HAR
IN MY JESUS YEAR
REBECCA WOLFF

To make a long story short
I got no sleep

Mid-nighttime visitation to the thrashing
body. Only after the question is asked
do we see a presupposition

sprawled out like a cat:

gloom is terrifying
comes with its own font
a dose of cremation

in the chamber
set on constant agitation
You see me not only at my worst

but in the grips
of an exalted digression
Rainspot

rainspot
the streets will be rinsed
clean in the morning but I dare

not go visit them.
With only my body to express
intention

My mind to confer
character

and the threat or treat of sunspot.
Put my cap on:
I escape that bad night

and set my cap for—
put a cap on . . .

You start doing it
and then you learn you are in
the grand tradition:

Holy terror
all my life I had asked for
an inarguable

treatment
like Alice James did
white sheet

in the black
carapace.
Who are you that stands around and shakes

who are you that rolls the waves
who are you that steals cool
from the air and crafts fear for me.

TUESDAY

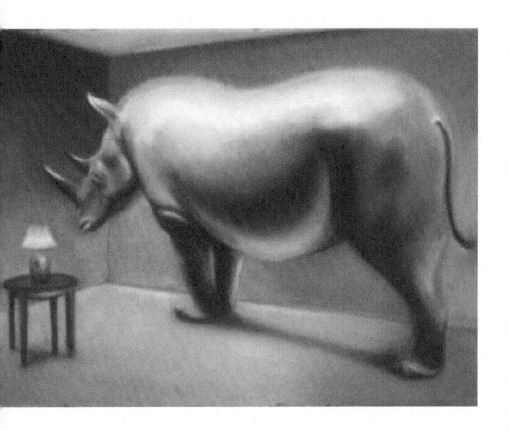

Sometimes a Massive Presence

CONTINUOUS THOUGHT
REBECCA WOLFF

It must have rained last night
the walk is puddled.

No single incident, but episodic
pouring

a drenching,
with intermittent silence
such that we could sleep through,
upstairs.

I slept through,
but in my sleep I guess I tried to speak

to describe a frequent
feeling.

When I can neither
sleep nor wake, when sleep
is full of all diseaseful matter
in solution: tall buildings
swaying unto death,
tall father's burnished reprimand × 10,
a muslin taste of not breathing, not ever again …

When I turn my head, is what I thought,
asleep, to say, but instead *"Every time …"*
is what I said. "Every time I open my mouth …"; then

AWAKE!
fell back down; apparently
you gave to me a sip of water. (Every time

I open my mouth and turn my head at the same time
my throat closes, a mechanism in a badly made,
overly ambitious doll,
one who never sleeps.)

Nothing in this single time.
I would not think to tell you of it
if it was not episodic.

TAKING OUT THE TRASH
PRISCILLA BECKER

I got a good night's sleep last night and that is partly why I am writing this essay, because my brain is not addled and at low tide. It's a rare feeling, at once a presence and an absence: the presence of my whole mind, the absence of the obscure and needling sense of disintegration.

I am refreshed, a feeling so uncommon it resembles fatigue—my natural state—my derelict receptors unable to recognize this new condition. It is as though a valve has been opened and, sensing the deep longed-for pleasure of sleep, my body is slowly leaking the whole of its exhaustion.

I often attribute my insomnia to a current life situation: troubled relationship, sadistic boss, etc. But in truth a succession of "current situations" can be traced back for as long as I can recall, about twenty-five years.

And I've had just as many theories about my insomnia's resolution: In my teens I was convinced I couldn't sleep because I wasn't skinny enough. The consequent twenty-year course of anorexia didn't clear things up. Besides, often I would wake from a nightmare in which I'd eaten several Big Macs; in my twenties I decided what I needed was a warm body beside me. It took a long while for me to recognize this theory as the theory of promiscuity that it was, and not a solution of insomnia. Next a theory of physical tension developed. This tension demanded its release through yoga. My dedication to yoga obscured obligations to family and career. It also defied sense, and sometimes I would wake in the night in fear that I would not be able to conform my work schedule to my yoga practice. Next came a subset of the yoga theory: inversions in the morning would stimulate my system during the day, while inversions at night would stimulate my system at night. So I spent a good amount of energy worrying over my schedule of flipping my legs in the air.

I offer the above as only an outlining of the course of manipulations I've subjected myself to over the years in an effort to solve my sleeplessness.

After a recent theory, dictating my going to bed by eleven, came to naught—for

AWAKE!

I found myself nervously adjusting my lifestyle around this tolling of the bell only to find that my inner insomniac smelled a rat and evened things out by waking me earlier in the morning—I have arrived at my latest theory, involving the trash.

Trash has long bothered me. Household trash, that is (though I sometimes also despair of the trash spilling over into the street, or the trash yachts sailing up and down the Hudson). I can't seem to leave it alone, in its receptacle, harming no one, disturbing nothing, for it plays on my psyche like a bad dream.

I have five waste baskets—one for each room. I cannot tell if I've just now disclosed something odd or typical. All I know is I have placed a basket in each of my rooms because I used to have just one—in the kitchen. I would find myself compelled to carry each scrap of paper, errant sock fuzz, or unidentifiable particle to the kitchen, interrupting any activity to do so. If I were eating and noticed a dust bunny settled in a corner of the room, I could not enjoy my meal until I'd picked it up and carried it to the trash; if I were having sex and felt a bump below my partner's back, I could not relax until I'd disposed of the offending granule; and most bothersome of all are the constant shedding strands of hair I encourage from my scalp by continually running my hands over the ends of my hair in order to feel if any have come loose: some always have. Of course I cannot simply allow these invisible fibers to float to the floor.

And so my remedy for my frequent trips to the kitchen was to place receptacles in each room, thus cutting down my travel time. What I did not foresee, however, was my equal compulsion toward consolidation, for if you were to peer into any but the kitchen trash, you would find nothing there.

And the reason for this is that I do not use these secondary receptacles. Occasionally I will place something in one of them, only to remove it soon afterward, delivering it to its mother, the kitchen trash. This I carry almost daily to the trash courtyard on the ground floor of my building.

My apartment is constructed like the sun: there is a central room from which four other rooms emanate like rays. It is possible for me to see three of the five receptacles from my main perch in this focal room. I can feel surrounded.

This fear is not, I don't think, what it may seem: I do not have nightmares about expanding trash, nor am I any sort of germ-a-phobe. Accumulation of any kind does however tend to make me unhappy: I like to throw things out. I can do this with aplomb, sometimes without even looking. I do not lack sentimentality, though I will throw out your letters.

If you are getting the idea that I am fanatically orderly, that I set the papers on my desk flush to its border and face all the fronts of my shirts hanging in my closet to the east, you would be mistaken, for my compulsion seems to have its specific fixation in trash.

Most often when I wake in the night, it is with the sense that there is something I have forgotten to do, an acute yet obscure dread, for when I try to name what it is I should be doing, nothing definitive pierces my mind. I can, however, think of a long list of things I should do more of or pay more attention to, vast unfulfilled dreams, or neglected but not pressing tasks. Why these vague chores and dreams that during the day do not rouse me to any action should wake me in the night with a sense of urgency, though, I do not know.

From an early age I was a budding insomniac, and my mother's condition was in full flower. She had a habit of playing the piano in the middle of the night. The music would waft up the stairs and under my closed door, arriving transformed—muffled, a little sour-sounding. I pictured a madman at the organ, pounding away in the cellar of a derelict mansion. This gothic sense was heightened by the framed photograph of my dead maternal grandfather placed on top of the piano: he looked like Vincent Price. My other grandfather looked like Hitler, but that is another story, I think.

As a child I had supersonic hearing. I mention this not because it would have taken any to detect my mother's playing, but because I've posited it from time to time as another of my theories of insomnia. I am also unusually responsive to light. Just the suggestion of it when attempting to sleep makes me recoil, like a reverse photosynthesis.

But it has always eluded me whether my hearing was innate or evolved due to a condition of my upbringing: my mother had to have us (my sister and me) completely at her disposal. She had a special call she'd let loose that meant that we were to come running. It was a two-note soprano song distinctive throughout the neighborhood as some kind of "Becker girl round-up". She'd sound her pitch and then drop down a major third. She used it to call my sister and me whether we were outside in the neighborhood or inside the house. The sound embarrassed me: none of the other children suffered such special treatment. It also filled me with fear.

My mother's temper is extraordinary. If we did not hear or heed her call, instantly materializing in defiance of time and space logic, an anger that deepened with each passing moment would be touched off. I would hear her round-up song and leave whatever I was doing mid-stream: drop my book, bounding down the stairs; abandon my wandering the empty plot next door, tearing toward home.

AWAKE!

There were many accompanying provisos. For instance I was not allowed to listen to rock music. I had a stereo, however, a circular black and silver apparatus that had a clear round plastic dust cover and looked like a spaceship, on which I was permitted to play my classical LP's. Unknown to my parents, I had a modest collection of rock records as well—KISS and Peter Frampton, Cheap Trick, etc, which I hid between the covers of my classical records.

My method for listening to them was as follows: I'd "borrow" my mother's gigantic brown headphones from her living room stereo, sneaking them into my room. My mother was often to be heard screaming in exasperation whenever she'd notice them missing. I'd lie on my bedroom floor, put the headphones on, making certain that the sound was not escaping through the room speakers. I'd angle one of the ears of the headphones away from me and slightly off my ear, which split my stereo experience down the middle. But it also lent me ambient access—the reason for this contortion. Then I'd crank the sound.

When I heard my mother's two-note song, my hand, which hovered by the panel of knobs, would instantly switch the stereo off. I'd dash down the stairs, presenting myself to her within seconds, for it was not enough just to answer: the first note of her call was a reveille, the second, an alarm.

I was not allowed to watch TV either—another craving I gratified whenever I sensed the opportunity. I would stand close to the screen with the sound turned very low, ready to slam it off at the hint of enemy approach.

In any case, my hearing either evolved or was given to me at birth, the gods perhaps sensing my special need. My sister, however, has no such "gift," for she developed other methods of coping with our home life. It is a dubious dispensation in any event: the sound of a dog's bark is painful to me, and, though I love riding a bike, I ride in fear that a car will honk its horn, startling me to my death.

As an adult I have worked to lessen the perception of my ears, attending thousands of rock shows, where I stand directly in front of the speakers. I've met with some success: the edge has been burned off my hearing.

On Saturday mornings my sister and I would wake—early: there was no option of sleeping in—to a list of chores scrawled in my mother's illegible hand, as though one of the furies had touched down in the night. There was evidence of a very long base list to which new insights had been added haphazardly, protruding from the original like angry tentacles.

The duties that belonged to us were the cleaning of the whole house (I won't belabor the lawn mowing, two and a half acres, which we were also responsible for, but whose dispensation was the provenance of my father)—thirteen rooms, counting staircase and hallways. For the "living" rooms, this cleaning meant basically vacuuming and dusting. My mother liked to give tutorials about moving all the furniture to access the secret pockets of dirt lurking in dark corners. There was also one on dusting, a three-process chore.

The species of room in which food was ingested or expelled from the body had special considerations, and we were trained to scrub mildew from the grouting surrounding each tile that lined the showers from the edge of the bathtubs to the ceilings. The wood cabinets of the kitchen had to be cleaned and oiled; the counters and stove, bordered by stainless steel, purged of their wet black grime using toothpicks.

And I'm not sure I have the spirit to go into my mother's special projects.

My sister would set right in on her chores and by afternoon was free to do something of her choosing, at least theoretically. But my response was paralysis, and I would spend the day sitting on my bed trying in vain to will myself to action, leaping to a mockery of it whenever my mother approached. My immobility was thorough; even my respiration would slow.

I was plagued by an episode of The Little Rascals, watched illicitly, in which the diminutive gang glues a bunch of babies left in their charge to the floor. The babies cry and try to rip their bottoms from the floor, but to no avail. I thought often of these babies rendered helpless by the will of another. The episode also excited me sexually. But that is another story, I think.

In any case, my day of freedom would chug by, each minute stretched painfully. But I was not rewarded for my stamina, for what I did not complete one day would be commuted to the next. As a result, my duties would accumulate and punishments accrue, making my activity seldom. I was only set free on those rare and fortunate days when I could summon the energy to reconfigure enough of the domestic tableau to pass inspection. A curiosity of my mother's nature is that she is both overbearing and neglectful, and it was possible, though uncommon, that the appearance of these characteristics would fall into the proper alignment, and I could get away with something.

But most often I was in a slow-dawning sort of trouble, and over the course of the day and night my mother would discover that I'd done nothing. Sometimes then she would shake me awake in the night. I would be disoriented and frightened, sure that my father had died or the house was on fire. She would hover above me saying my name. I remember the strange sort of fear—part dread, part comfort at having my mother so near.

When I fully came to, my mother's face would be very close to mine, her arms around my back, her green eyes piercing me with the intensity of her rage. She would command me from my bed, downstairs and into the kitchen where my punishment was waiting for me: the full receptacle of trash.

This is the middle-night rendezvous I remember best. But there were others—a rag or broom in my mother's hand.

Dressed in my nightgown, I would carry the trash outside and set it by the side of the road. I remember walking back very slowly and peering down the empty street.

I wasn't in any rush to return to bed. My sister would probably be awake, watching me with that look that early on characterized the nature of her sisterly gaze: part pity, part fear, part elation at the rewards of her skill for avoidance of trouble. I never quite knew if I'd been sacrificed.

She claims that more often I'd watch her: our beds were arranged in an L-shape, and from the perch of my headboard, many nights I'd stare down at her sleeping form. My staring would make her awaken. I remember her mild irritation—she seemed more perplexed than annoyed. But because she was older, and her disgust with me de rigueur, she feigned a sort of anger.

These were nice moments between us, when our eyes would meet and she'd whine out my name: *Pris*, she'd say, dragging her abbreviation of my name into two syllables: *What is your problem? Why aren't you sleeping?*

DO SCIENTISTS DREAM OF SLEEPLESS SHEEP?

MOLLY KOTTEMANN

I doubt that the sleep of a scientist is much different from that of a writer, a painter, a helmsman. Although my dreams of work often consist of the gaga green curves of fluorescent fly brains more so than desks or palettes or tillers, when I sleep, I sleep much like any other slumberer. We are all the same, when we sleep, brain waves like hurdy-gurdys droning us down; we are all sunk deep into the same inscrutable landscape. It is when the scientist cannot sleep that the differences arise, diaphanous but discrete, like soap-bubbles. I have listened to the complaints of other insomniacs, noting their particular patterns, tracing their pathways of non-sleep. Listening, I have heard accounts of a dreadful grey half-consciousness, or of constant attention to the things one could be doing, must be doing, turn on the lights right now, there are dishes to be washed! When I cannot sleep, I neither lie in listless limbo nor construct pyramids of teetering needs and failures on the verge of collapse. When I cannot sleep, my thoughts aching but strangely lucid, I curl sullen in my sheets and think about why.

The scientific notion of sleep is couched in jargon, more mechanism than metaphor, but remains nearly as mysterious as its poetic counterpart. As we begin to ravel its knitted sleeve, it eludes us with ever more knots. We now know the brain region that controls our circadian rhythms—the suprachiasmatic nucleus, a word that for me conjures much more than its anatomical etymology and conveys an aetherial organizer that resides above the intersection of sleep and waking. We have identified elements of the genome that regulate the expression of the proteins and hormones that dictate these cycles, elements that are heavily conserved from humans down to tiny flatworms, underscoring the fundamental mechanisms that have arisen from living in this twenty-four hour rhythm of light and dark. We can approximate the neurochemistry that signals our brains to adjust its patterns and lull us into somnolence. Still, the acres of papers and narcoleptic fruit flies aside, we lie abed, pressing seemingly lidless eyes and waiting for sleep to answer our insistent knocks.

AWAKE!

The suprachiasmatic nucleus (SCN), a bit of brain tissue within the hypothalamus that contains only 20,000 neurons—a mere 0.00002% of the brain's complement—has been demonstrated to control circadian rhythms within the central nervous system. *Insane!* I sometimes mumble to myself at night. *How could such a minority wreak such havoc on my beleaguered brain?* For better or worse (*Worse!* that sleep-deprived voice interjects indignantly) the nervous system is no democracy: this tiny region effects its signals through glands that release hormones, like melatonin, that proscribe global brain patterns. Within the retina reside photoreceptors that, unlike the canonical rods and cones that cluster behind our eyes like traffic cones and posts arranged by an artful hooligan, do not contribute to vision, but rather transduce light stimuli to the SCN. Even blind marmosets can synchronize their circadian rhythm with light cues. The SCN, oneiric oligarch, integrates photic signals with a complex web of cellular crosstalk and cycles of protein synthesis and degradation to yield, ultimately and ideally, the flux of delicious drowsiness and piquant awakening so coveted by the tossing insomniac.

I myself have been known to rail against reductionism, often after a long stint in the laboratory and one too many brandies. It is uncomfortable when emotions are deconstructed into gene patterns, when we are told that the sensation of waking next to your love, a man with a mouth like mown grass and geodes, is a jigsaw of major histocompatability complexes and evolutionarily determined hormone patterns. And while sleep is surely no emotion, sleepless nights can acquire an existential immediacy that seems impossible to understand piecemeal, genes and dopamine. Yet even these can be traced back to molecular biology. There are many genes that have been implicated as playing roles on sleep's stage, named with alternating prosaicism and whimsy. There are the mouse genes *"Mop3"* and *"Clock,"* the *Drosophila* gene *"Timeless,"* the *Arabidopsis* gene *"Time for coffee."* Mutating *Mop3* in mice results in animals with abolished circadian rhythmicity: when deprived of light, they remain aimlessly active, running on their wheels in the darkness, lacking the phasic locomotion observed in their unmutated counterparts.

Circadian rhythm gene products, while embroiled in a complex ferment of cross-regulation, also regulate themselves in an Ouroborosian manner. As soon as a protein begins to accumulate in the cell, it initiates its own destruction, setting off branching messages that eventually wend their way back to the nucleus and tell the cell to cease its production, mechanisms that tag it for degradation. Tracing the rise and fall of these gene products reveals that they are impeccably timed to complete their circle within the space of twenty-four hours. Perhaps it is tiny permutations in this pathway that leave us stranded along the road to slumber.

Even plants, those verdant but sessile organisms with no nervous system to speak of, have circadian rhythms. Although it is at first strange to ascribe this quality, this phenomenon that seems so tangibly and specifically human those nights I lie in bed, stubbornly and endlessly awake, to the African violet that sits placid and furry on my windowsill, it is not, upon reflection, surprising. It is not, upon reflection, difficult to imagine some insomniacal morning glory, twined around a trellis with its petals still stubbornly open against the night. And despite the anthropomorphization I indulge in during those nights, the inscrutable ticking of molecular clocks has been logically and rigorously characterized in *Arabidopsis thaliana*, the gangly weed embraced by plant geneticists.

Scientists have found numerous regulatory elements in the *Arabidopsis* genome that control the peaks and troughs in gene expression that are coupled to the sidereal day. The actions of these elements may be viscerally visualized by placing a reporter gene—a gene that produces a trackable response—under their control. Eerily, this reporter is often luciferase, the chemical that produces the unearthly glow in the abdomen of the nychthemeral firefly, causing the plants to luminesce along with the progression of their circadian cycles. Sometimes, during those nights, I imagine the light that rises and ebbs inexorably within the tissues of such plants, letting the soft and lambent pulse draw me back into my own rhythm of sleep and waking.

I doubt that the sleep of a scientist is much different from that of a writer, a painter, a helmsman. But when I, a scientist, cannot, I take a certain comfort in the fact that I and my fellow forgers of fact are the archaeologists of sleep, slowly chipping away at the stubborn bedrock that surrounds its skeleton. I take a certain comfort in naming the stepping stones in our stream of study. Rather than counting sheep, cataloguing colors, imagining flying fish leaping in sedative sequence, I speak their names to myself. *Mop3*, I murmur. *Clock, time for coffee, timeless. timeless. timeless.* And sometimes, even this promise of knowledge lulls me down into dream.

DAWN OF THE DEAD
NEAL POLLACK

Insomnia hits me about once a month, maybe twice. On those dread nights, no amount of dull-book-reading, ESPN Classic-watching, or desperate pre-dawn masturbation sessions can relax the rabbit thump of my heart, which increases in speed and intensity with every ten-minute turnover of the clock. As the low-lying panic sets in, my worried thoughts tend to turn toward the usual subjects that plague insomniacs: that bill I should have paid, that phone call I should have made, what I should have said to that guy about that thing, basketball statistics, and my perception of the rising or declining stock of my literary reputation. Perhaps that last one is unique to me. Still, I understand the mind of the insomaniacal person.

However, despite the ordinary topics that take over my mind on sleepless nights, the root cause of my insomnia is, I think, somewhat different from the average. I work at home, with irregular hours. In fact, my hours are so irregular that no one except me (and, for some reason, my father) cares whether or not I work at all. This means a late start to the workday, 10 a.m., noon, 6 p.m., whenever, and it also means that I don't have to get up to go to work in the morning. Most people my age (the back end of the mid-thirties) stopped sleeping in long ago. I, on the other hand, cling to that vestige of bohemian privilege with an ironclad will and a broad collection of earplugs. Sleeping is fun. Nothing wakes me up in the morning.

That said, occasionally I have to get up before sunrise. There are few things that can cause this to occur, but those things do sometimes come down the pike. I have an early flight. I have . . . actually, early flights are pretty much it these days, other than some family circumstances that I'll delineate later. But the nights when I cannot sleep are still fairly rare, which is good, because my need to have a daily lie-in looms so great that the mere thought of having to get up at 4:30 a.m. fills me with a dread unto death. Therefore, I know in advance that whenever I have to wait in line so I don't end up getting a middle seat on a morning cross-country Southwest flight from Baltimore to Austin, I'll be very tired. I know that if I have to get up at dawn, then I'm going to end up seeing dawn from both ends.

*

Anticipating your own exhaustion is exhausting in itself. Sometimes, I think that I'd rather be dead than tired. At least when you're dead, you don't have to get up in the morning. But it hasn't been like this my entire life. As a boy, I routinely got up at 5:30 a.m. to watch cartoons. In high school, my alarm went off at 6 a.m. every weekday, not because I needed to get up quite that early, but because I wanted to hear an unsubtle sports comedy segment on the local Morning Zoo that I found hilarious. The name of the sports comedian was Cookie "Chainsaw" Randolph, and he was an all-American doofus of the highest order, as well as, so he claimed, Steve Garvey's illegitimate half-brother. I'm stunned to discover, as I Google his name now, that the Cookster is still working, and is, in fact, the sports guy for the highest-rated morning show in San Diego. I guess some guys are better at working a one-note shtick into a long career than others. Crazy.

But back to the essay at hand: even in college, where every non-pre-med coed slumbers during the day like a concubine of Nosferatu, I regularly scheduled 8 a.m. and 9 a.m. classes for myself. At some point, though, I found myself dropping out for three-hour afternoon naps. I found myself sleeping until 3 on Sundays. And then I graduated from college, and I just kept on sleeping.

I'm not delivering an epistle for laziness. On occasion, I've been known to work. There are books, magazine articles, and pieces in anthologies like this one that prove my output hasn't been completely stunted by late sleeping. I'm just saying that when I'm forced to get up, or even to get dressed, my work suffers, because that's when the night terrors beset me. Fortunately, I found my first full-time job at the only newspaper in the world that doesn't want its reporters to come into the office, ever. This was a newsweekly in Chicago that operated under the foolish theory that reporters could come up with better stories if they weren't gossiping in the newsroom all the time. In my case, I never found a story that began before noon.

For the rare stories where circumstances forced me to interview a person who only had time for me before breakfast, I suffered all night long. One morning at age twenty-five, after having fallen asleep at 3:30 a.m. and woken up at 4:30 a.m., I took the El to the near South Side to meet a Cadillac-driving ghetto lawyer who vaguely resembled Bernie Casey in alligator shoes. I could barely focus on the road ahead as this lawyer and I drove two hours to Dixon, Illinois, and could barely form questions with my furry tongue while he extolled to me the many virtues of his misunderstood client, Gangster Disciples boss Larry Hoover.

Thus it came to pass that I interviewed one of the most powerful criminals in America while in an insomnia-induced brain fog. The resulting story did nothing to rehabilitate his reputation, which is good, because as it turns out he set up a "save the children" fund in order to launder drug money, a time-honored Chicago tradition practiced by black and white alike. Why do I bring this up now? Because I hate getting up in the morning so much that I remember every incident of insomnia. For instance, I vividly recall having insomnia one night in November 1996. I had to get up early to receive an award for helping return a semi-retarded adult man to his elderly mother after he'd been held prisoner in a Wisconsin nursing home for months. The exhaustion I felt the next day still haunts me, unhealthily.

*

After I quit my newspaper job, morning professional obligations ceased almost entirely. When I read about authors who say they do their best work before 9 a.m., I think two things: they're lying, or they're suckers. What's the point of being a professional writer if you can't sleep late most of the time? But the last few years have brought new challenges, as far as sleeping in goes. On October 31, 2002, I became a father. Having a young child defeats even the strongest sleepers.

On the predetermined mornings when my wife gets to sleep in and I have to get up with the kid, I rise between 6 and 7 a.m. after having stayed up until 3 or 4 a.m. I'll go to bed at 10 or 11 with the best of intentions and sometimes will even find myself in that pleasant drifting state just before unconsciousness reigns. Then my fear of dawn kicks in, and suddenly, I can't stop thinking about the trades the Dodgers made this offseason, or my health-insurance payments, or, inevitably, all matters sexual. Usually, a bout of insomnia covers all these topics and then some. Then the kid is awake and I'm on the sofa, blanket drawn over my head, while he bathes in the warm multicultural corporate glow of *Dora the Explorer* and its boy-geared spinoff, *Go Diego Go!*

By noon, I'm bumping into walls.

"I have to lie down," I say to my wife.

"What's the point of you getting up with him early if you just end up taking a three-hour nap in the afternoon?" she says.

"I've got to make up that sleep somehow."

"Can't you just wait until he goes to bed? Please? I need you to hang in there."

"No."

Sometimes, though, she ends up guilting me into staying up all day. I hit multiple plateaus of exhaustion, and usually drop things. I find myself nodding off in the car, jarred awake by a pinch on the thigh. Then, eventually, the kid is in bed and I'm free. The next morning's sleep spreads before me like the wide-open *pampas*. Because of that, I can stay up as late as I want. So on days when I can sleep in, the converse happens. I stay up until 2 because I know that 10 a.m. awaits me on the other side.

If even the worst insomniac got to sleep late once in a while, insomnia wouldn't be much of a problem, because insomnia isn't really about not being able to sleep at night. It's about not being able to sleep until noon. I realize the following is low on the list of necessary social reforms, but it's one I wholeheartedly support: if the world just started a few hours later, we wouldn't be talking about insomnia anymore. For the sake of humankind, and especially for me, let's all work together to make it so.

INSOMNI-WHACK
JONATHAN AMES

First there was a homosexual fantasy. It happens whenever I'm low on money. I feel weak, humiliated, pathetic, so then I see an erect organ, not my own, presenting itself. What follows is an imagined moment of cruel sensuality. Then the thought: it would probably hurt. And then I think about disease. By now the whole fantasy is shot, so I'm just sort of beat round the head by the thing or it stares at me in a menacing way. Then I'm reaching for the hand towel, which I've hidden under my pillow, and cleaning up the unfortunate mess.

It's the same fantasy every time with very little change; it all occurs in a shadowy void, though once in a while there's a prison cell as a backdrop. Last night it happened, and, as always, I regretted the whole thing. But I am weak, weak. Always giving in. I've been destroying my body and my mind and my hair and my soul with masturbation for eighteen years. I'm wasting away. People often say to me: you're so thin. It's because I'm on a steady diet of jerking off. I wonder if it would work for women. I could become rich. Solve my money problems. Write a book encouraging women to lose weight through masturbation.

I tried to fight the urge last night, but I did it because I thought it would help me sleep. And I need sleep. Four nights in a row, I've had terrible, relentless insomnia. It is a symptom of my growing depression, which, like the homosexual fantasies, has been brought on by my financial troubles. Somehow I was doing all right in '97, probably because I received my advance for my second novel, but I've gone through the whole thing, and it wasn't much, and now everything's fallen apart here in early '98. I've paid my January rent, but that's it. Haven't paid the phone bill, electric bill, health insurance, minimum charges on maxed-out credit cards with interest rate at 21 percent, and now I'm getting letters and phone calls about making payments on my enormous graduate school loans. And I don't even remember going to graduate school. It was a three-year drunken blur in the early nineties resulting in a useless degree. It couldn't possibly be worth fifty thousand dollars.

The whole thing is crushing, debilitating. And like all of my problems, it's entirely my fault. So I'm depressed, defeated, morbid, *and* I have insomnia. Each night I've woken up at 4 a.m. The first night I felt like my whole life was a lie—the kind of thought one has at that hour; the second night I kept saying to myself, Maybe I should just die; and the third night I was resigned and less full of self-pity and I read a whole *New York Press* and the first two chapters of *The Brothers Karamazov*.

Then last night, even after the masturbation, I slept for only a few hours and again woke up at 4 a.m. I pretended that I must be thirsty and I took a drink from the water bottle next to my bed. Then I closed my eyes. Snuggled against the pillow. But I couldn't fool the insomnia demons. They knew I wasn't parched. Oh, God, I'm up again, I thought. To try to fall back to sleep I played two of my usual hero fantasies through my head: (1) I save a woman from rape, but I am stabbed by the assailant, though I still manage to knock him unconscious. The police and EMS arrive and I'm rushed to a hospital. I survive, and the next day I'm hailed as a hero on the front pages of the tabloids: WRITER SAVES WOMAN. (2) I wake up one day with incredible jumping powers and I get a tryout with the Knicks, make the team, and I'm hailed on the *back* pages: 5' 11" 33-YEAR-OLD WRITER CAN DUNK!

But I was too depressed to really work up the hero stories and fill them with pleasurable details, so I turned on the light and saw the Dostoyevsky, but couldn't face it, the long names. So I read two Graham Greene short stories. The names are easier. And then I was too tired to read anymore, but it wasn't the kind of tired that lets you sleep. That kind of tired is like a book closing gently; insomnia tired is like the pages of the book are slowly burning, curling inward, turning black. There's no rest, just the torture of nerves coming undone, fraying.

So then I started to whack off again. I was hoping that two sessions in a four-hour span would put me out. This time the fantasy was heterosexual. I thought of this unnamed beauty whom I often see on Second Avenue. I imagined us talking on the street. I say to her, "I've seen you for months. I find you very beautiful." She invites me up to her apartment. She lies on her bed. She's naked. My head is between her legs, she pulls me in tight, my nose is inside her. I cry and weep and take comfort in her delicious womb. Then the thought intrudes: Since I've picked her up on the street, she probably hasn't had a chance to shower for a few hours and maybe she'll have a bad urine smell. I don't judge her for this, but what if it's genuinely unpleasant? I push this thought out of my mind, but I seem to take heed in my fantasy. I rise up from her pussy and her arms are over her head. The full bounty of her breasts is revealed to me. I pounce. We join. Splendor. Enchantment. Rapture. I reach for the towel.

AWAKE!

The whole thing, like the homoerotic masturbating session, lasted about forty-five seconds. I never give myself any foreplay. I've been prematurely ejaculating while masturbating for years. The images come lightning fast, and then I come lightning fast. As soon as it's over, I don't remember if there was any pleasure. It happens too quick. Also the thing must be worn out like an old needle on a record player. There's probably not much sensitivity left. Masturbation, for me, has become purely a nervous habit, like cracking my knuckles.

I was hoping at least that it would help me sleep—two debilitating releases in four hours—but no, I was wide awake and yet exhausted. I got dressed and decided that I would go to the Kiev and pollute myself with an enormous sleep-inducing meal.

It was 5 a.m. I trudged up deserted, freezing Second Avenue. I felt limp-dicked from the masturbating. My nostrils burned from the cold. My beautiful woman was asleep somewhere. The avenue was sort of lovely in its emptiness. I bought a *Post*.

Paula Jones was on the cover, and I was saddened. I love Clinton. I once dreamt that he said to me, "You're going to be all right," and it was very reassuring. And I don't care if he's libidinous. Alpha males—leaders—are supposed to be that way. I'm a *zeta male* and *I'm* sex-crazed, so I can imagine that the sex drive at the top of the alphabet must be unbearable.

I went into the Kiev and an adorable, light-haired Polish waitress approached with a menu. "Good morning," she said. "How are you?" Her smile was real, endearing.

"Lousy," I said. "Insomnia." But she was already walking away from me, not listening. I wanted her to mother me. I want all beautiful waitresses to mother me. And they are like mothers—the good ones; they're sweet to you and they bring you food. Just two nights ago, I borrowed some money from a friend and went into a Thai restaurant and ordered a bowl of soup. These two Thai waitresses, with beautiful exposed arms, were so solicitous. I didn't deserve such kindness, I felt. If I could have a harem, I'd compose it with all the beautiful waitresses I've known and worshipped.

I studied the Kiev menu. I decided to get the Breakfast Sampler. It was weighty and noxious: ten slices of kielbasa, bacon, krakus ham, a single pancake, and a piece of French toast. I was raised kosher and I hardly ever eat pork except when I'm feeling self-destructive.

The waitress-angel floated back over. "How's the Sampler?" I asked.

"It's good," she said in her delightful singsong Polish accent.

"What's krakus ham?" I asked. "Is it from Krakow? Is it Polish for carcass?"

She smiled at me. She spoke English well, but nothing I was saying made sense to her. "Do you want coffee?" she asked.

"Oh, no," I said. "I have insomnia."

She looked at me tenderly. I could have kissed her. She walked away. I imagined her hiding me out during the war years in her barn. She'd bring me krakus ham. We'd make love. I'd survive the war and she and I would come to America and open up the Kiev. I was delirious.

My food came. I ate, and I read the sports section. There was another article on my new hero, Keith Van Horn. I can't help it—I do root for white basketball players. I ate all the pork and found that it was waking me up. All the nitrates in the meat must have been energizing me. I stayed in the Kiev until 6:30. I paid my bill—it was all of $4.87. I left a dollar tip, like a valentine.

I stepped outside. The sun was up. I was wide awake. I walked down Second Avenue. It wasn't so lovely anymore. Vulturish taxis filled the road. I trudged home. I came in and a cockroach jogged across the floor. I though of Kafka, which made me think of writing. I sat down at my desk and wrote, "First there was a homosexual fantasy."

A LITTLE NIGHT MISERY

HOWARD CRUSE

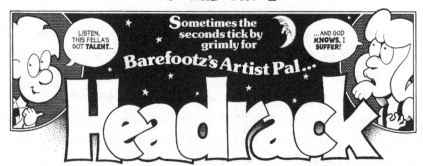

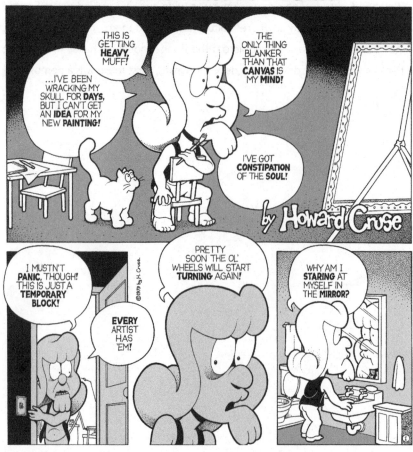

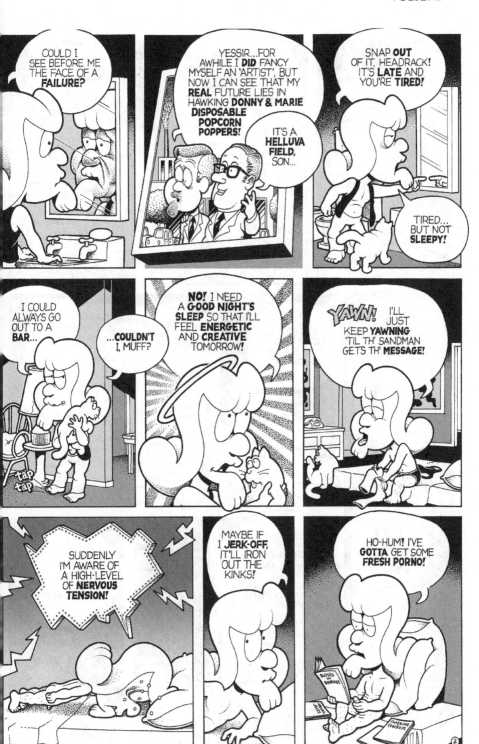

97

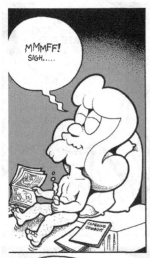

MMMFF! SIGH.....

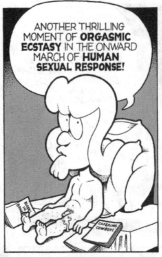

ANOTHER THRILLING MOMENT OF **ORGASMIC ECSTASY** IN THE ONWARD MARCH OF **HUMAN SEXUAL RESPONSE!**

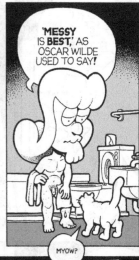

'MESSY IS **BEST,'** AS OSCAR WILDE USED TO SAY!

MYOW?

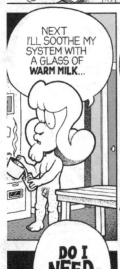

NEXT I'LL SOOTHE MY SYSTEM WITH A GLASS OF **WARM MILK...**

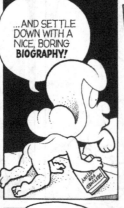

...AND SETTLE DOWN WITH A NICE, BORING **BIOGRAPHY!**

didn't have long to wait. The genius of the young artist was quickly recognized, and wealthy buyers flocked to his studio.

Freed forever from worries about food and rent, the busy 19-year-old was able to dedicate himself even m̶ fervently to the pursuit of his uniq̶ ̶ion, which swiftly became̶ celebrated throughou̶ civilized world.

"I guess you might̶ lucky," he re̶̶ interview wi̶ "My artistic i̶ plus the sexua̶ ful̶̶

DESTINED FOR DESTINY

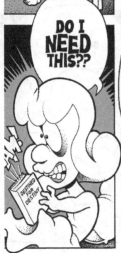

DO I **NEED** THIS??

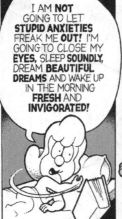

I AM **NOT** GOING TO LET **STUPID ANXIETIES** FREAK ME **OUT!** I'M GOING TO CLOSE MY **EYES**, SLEEP **SOUNDLY**, DREAM **BEAUTIFUL DREAMS** AND WAKE UP IN THE MORNING **FRESH** AND **INVIGORATED!**

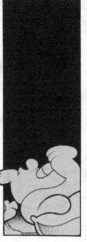

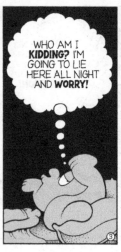

WHO AM I **KIDDING?** I'M GOING TO LIE HERE ALL NIGHT AND **WORRY!**

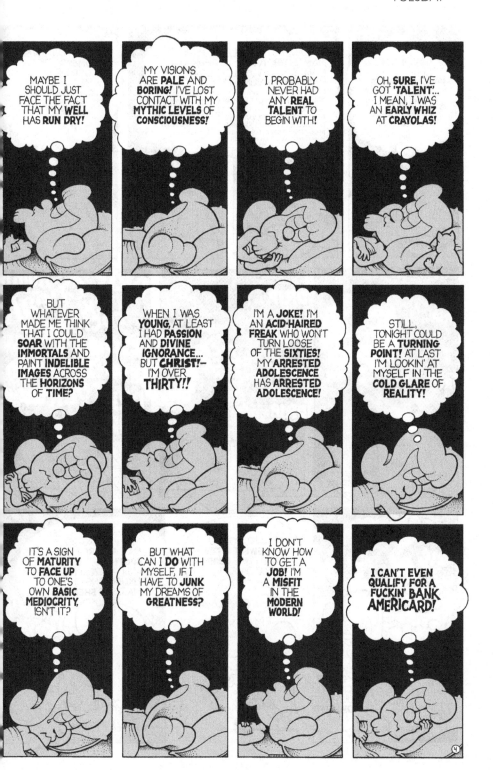

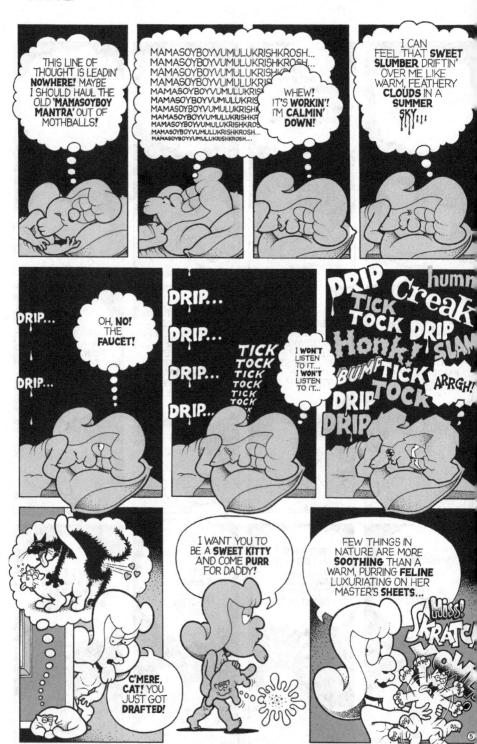

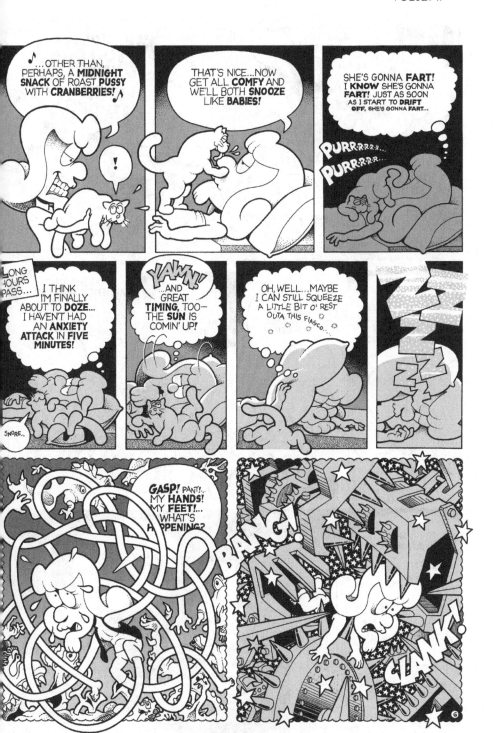

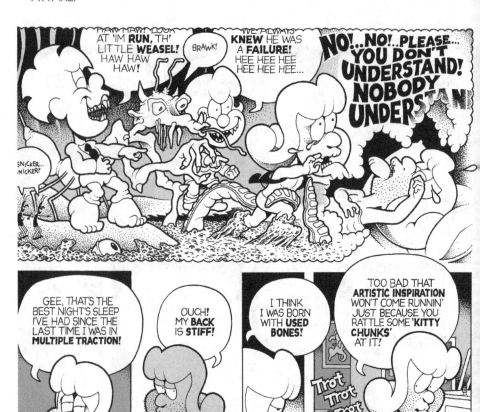

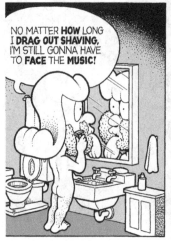

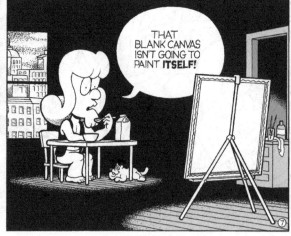

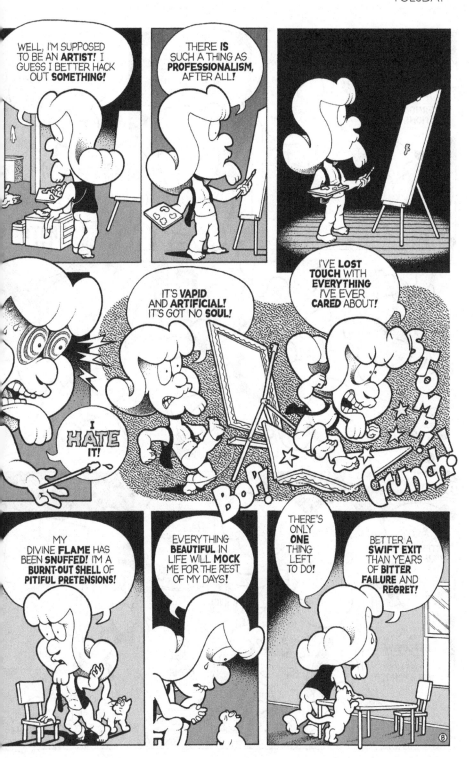

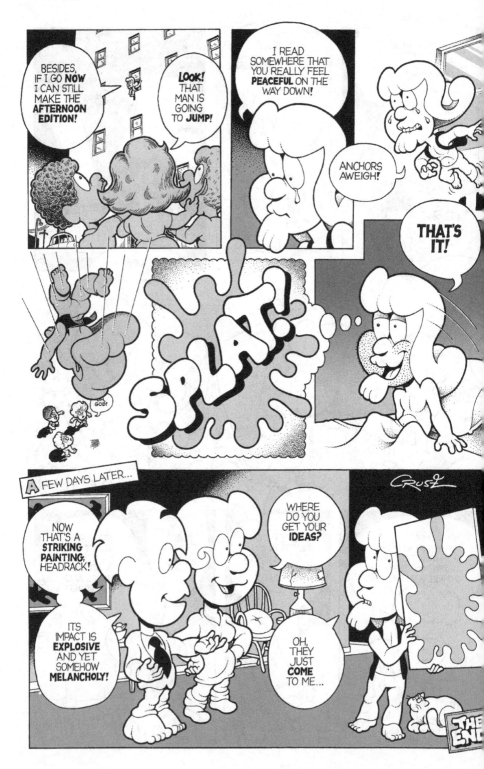

LINCOLN, ARISEN

STEVE ALMOND

Sleep hath its own world.

—Byron

On March 14, 1865, with the war drawn to a close and the cherry trees budding, Lincoln dispatches Under Secretary Dole to convey a message along to Douglass, inviting him to take tea at the Soldier's Home.

Douglass removes the sheet of foolscap from its dainty envelope. His hair, which in official portraits will take the appearance of a bald eagle perching atop his head, dips toward his brow. "Is this a prank, Dole?"

"No sir. The President requests your company."

"My company?"

"I should think that apparent."

Douglass frowns. Nearby, a clock tolls six. He looks about in agitation. "But I have an engagement this evening, a speech."

"I see." Dole turns back to his carriage.

"I haven't time to cancel, sir. A hall has been rented; tickets issued." Rather too ardently, Douglass grasps Dole's sleeve. "Don't you see? I should be most honored to take tea with our beloved President. It is only this duty which compels me . . ."

Dole glances dubiously at Douglass's hand and nods to his driver.

"Perhaps on another occasion!" Douglass says. He is now half jogging alongside the carriage. "Perhaps—"

"Of course," murmurs Dole, as Douglass watches his hand draw the curtain shut.

*

Lincoln is tired of nobility. It has been years since he felt a single breeze of contentment. This he blames on nobility. Rectitude exhausts his every part. Days wash past in a torrent of reports and decisions. He peers at memoranda by lamplight,

AWAKE!

until the letters dance about like pickaninnies. At night, strange dreams press themselves upon him. Upon waking, he glances about his darkened bedroom and feels dread settling onto his skin like black damp.

I was happy once, he thinks: what on earth has happened?

*

"So this is the famous Mississippi?"

Lincoln nods, levers the flatboat toward the soft current at the river's center. They have just passed Red Wing.

His companion snorts.

"Yes?"

"I should have thought it wider."

"Give her a chance, Douglass. Rivers must be given a chance."

*

Senator Pomeroy escorts Douglass to the executive wing. Lincoln is in the antechamber to his office, on hands and knees, rooting among papers scattered on the floor. Pomeroy coughs discreetly. Lincoln rises, his legs seeming to unfold then unfold again, until he towers over Pomeroy, whose face shines like a small pink seashell.

"Mr. President," Pomeroy says, "may I present—"

"I know who he is, Senator." A forelock droops over Lincoln's eyes. He quietly bids the others from the room and sets a hand on Douglass's shoulder. "Seward has told me all about you. Sit down. I am glad to see you."

For the next hour, Douglass conveys the concerns of his race regarding military pay, commendations, the treatment of those captured by Confederates. Lincoln issues a pledge here, a vague promise there. Each man's posture is stiff, cautious.

There is a lengthy silence during which, it seems to Douglass, the entirety of a December dusk fills the jalousie windows behind Lincoln's desk. "I have the sense we have met somewhere before," Lincoln says. "Somewhere without all of this." He gestures at the dark wainscoting of his office, the massive leather chairs.

*

Lincoln takes his shoes off and cuffs his trousers. His tufted, coppery feet give him the appearance of a forest thing, an ogre. He stares at Douglass. "Take off that ridiculous garb," he says. "It is hot enough to melt a rail tie."

Douglass unbuttons his waistcoat, untabs the collar, folds them crisply. He removes his cuff links—a gift from the New England Freedman Association—and scans the wooden deck, shading his eyes. "Have you no chiffarobe?"

*

Douglass in Faneuil Hall. He stares at the puff pastry brought to him by Garrison. The cream of the abolitionist movement swirls around him: young men in golden spectacles, women in elaborate hoop dresses. Well-meaning folk agog at his capacity for speech. He pokes at the pastry, his finger sinking in. A great many people seem to want to talk to him at once.

"Douglass! Where is Douglass?"

"The proclamation's been issued!"

"Find Douglass!"

"Here he is. Speak Douglass! Speak!"

I am kept, Douglass thinks. As kept as china in an antique cabinet.

*

In a West Wing ceremony, Secretary of the Treasury Chase presents Lincoln with a newly minted twenty dollar bill. The president holds the note up to the light. "What a signature Mr. Spinner has," he says. "But it must take him hours to sign every bill. Tell me, how does he manage it?"

Chase lets out a laugh.

"What is funny, Chase?"

"Surely you realize, Mr. President."

"Realize what?"

"Spinner's signature, sir; it is engraved on the plate."

"*Engraved?*"

"Yes."

"What, then, is to keep a thief from stealing these plates? Or one of your staff from printing extras?"

Chase stares at him, unsure what to say. "But there are safeguards," he stammers.

Lincoln shakes his head. "This thing frightens me," he murmurs. "Not even our names are kept authentic any longer."

*

Lincoln rests his weight on the longpole, lets the boat drift. His eyes settle on Douglass. They are the color of bog peat. "Tell me about slavery."

"What is there to tell?" Douglass says impatiently. He is seated at his desk, endeavoring to compose his memoirs.

"What did you eat?"

"Cornbread. Salt pork. Whatsoever they gave us."

"When you say 'they'?"

Douglass continues scribbling. His plume bobs like a cock's wattle.

"And this talk of corporeal punishment, privations?"

Douglass offers no response.

Lincoln gazes out at the river, at the silvered eddies, and chuckles in a manner he hopes will provoke Douglass's interest. "I am reminded here of the one-legged Paducah planter. It seems he seeded his main acres with orchard rye, hoping to corner the market, leaving only a small patch for cotton. That season an early frost came, and our poor Paducah Joe was left without recourse—"

"Lincoln." Douglass holds his pen aloft. "If you might."

Lincoln gives his longpole a sullen yank.

"I rather like cornbread."

*

Douglass returns to the White House. Lincoln has aged a decade. His cheeks look like butcher paper, torn just beneath the eyes. "I have some concerns about the course of the conflict. Your people are not coming to us in the numbers I had hoped, Douglass." His tone is that of a peevish schoolmaster.

"They are trapped, Mr. President. Surely you can see."

"I want you to devise some way to bring them into our lines. Would you do that for me, Douglass? A band of scouts, perhaps?"

"I am hardly the man—"

"We will give you guns, Douglass. And rations and some pay."

"I very much doubt—"

"And morphine, Douglass. Morphine for the injured."

*

"How is it that you navigate this vessel?" Douglass says.

Lincoln has angled his body against the longpole. With his face upturned, his eyes closed, and the sun beating down, he looks, from this certain angle, like a large, sleepy turtle. "Navigate?" he says.

"Yes. Is there some rudder device, some means of control?"

Lincoln laughs. "The river is like history," he says. "And the flatboat is like a man's life. He can move about in the current, work the pole toward certain intended effects. But he is taken, finally, where river wishes to take him."

"And where is that, Mr. President?"

"To the sea, Douglass, the deep and final sea."

*

Lincoln's secretary pokes her head in the doorway. "Governor Buckingham of Connecticut," she says.

"Tell Governor Buckingham to wait," Lincoln snaps. "I want to have a long talk with my friend Frederick Douglass."

Douglass blushes. "Really, Mr. President. I am certain the Governor—"

"Hush, Douglass. I have no end of Buckinghams. That is why they keep me in this grand house. So the Buckinghams of the world know where to find me. Now then," Lincoln says, "we were discussing scouts. A band of them."

*

South of Burlington, Lincoln purchases a flask of whiskey from a passing gambling barge. Douglass, embarrassed, tries to hide beneath his desk.

"Say, is that Frederick Douglass?"

"No sir." Lincoln moves to shield his companion from view.

"Back away, you oaf. Let me see. But what other man could appear so Godawful? Look at his nose! Like a wedge of moldy cheese. Say there, Frederick!" Others now start to crowd the rail.

"I must ask you gentlemen to cease—"

"Is this your house nigger, Douglass?"

Lincoln steers away from the barge, but a crossflow drags them back.

"And where is Mrs. Douglass?"

"Come dance a waltz, Douglass."

"With your goon here. We've never before seen two niggers dance a waltz."

*

Disregarding the advice of his advisors, Lincoln invites a group of rail workers to the White House to celebrate the completion of a line to the Oregon territory. The men move about in rented waistcoats, a sea of nervous mustaches. Lincoln presses the men for accounts of the West. He is fascinated by buffalo, the talk of mountains and endless ridgelines. Long after the men have been marched off, Lincoln can be seen in the West Garden, his arms extended from his body, holding twelve-pound axes in either fist. He looks terribly sad planted there, like a scarecrow trembling in the wind.

*

Lincoln drops a cube of sugar in the flask and holds it out to Douglass.

"Thank you, no."

"Intemperance does you no favor, friend."

AWAKE!

"Still."

"As you wish." Lincoln swallows. "Tell me again about the good widow Glenwood, Douglass. Ah, now there was a woman who knew not to hide from virtue. And its tender erosions. Do not look upon me with such reproach, Douglass. It is not *I* who rhapsodizes my dreams. Also, I have found some sketches among your papers. I did not know you worked on the easel, Douglass."

"I do not."

Lincoln snorts with glee. "Good man! Have a nip!"

Douglass's cheeks redden. "Perhaps just a taste."

Lincoln stands and appears to wobble a bit. He snatches up his stovepipe, turns it onto his head. Sheaths of paper, stashed there with a pair of white kid gloves, flutter about. "What is all this rubbish?"

"You should keep your affairs at the desk," Douglass frets.

"How very important I am!" Lincoln cries, hopping about. "Coded dispatches from the front! Commendation order for one Corporal Bryce Riley! A speech in longhand!"

Douglass picks up the sheet at his feet. "What is this then?"

"How does it go?"

Douglass sniffs the flask and winces another swallow down. He clears his throat and reads: "'It may seem strange that any men should dare to ask a just God's assistance in wringing their bread from the sweat of other men's faces.'"

Lincoln shrugs. "Just a notion I've been playing with."

"Not bad, Lincoln. A bit tentative, perhaps."

Lincoln watches the wind hurl his papers, some landing on the rippled current. Others dance high in the golden noon, as if to drunkenly alight, before tangling in the bank's undergrowth. The merriment drains off Lincoln in dark sheets; his brow collapses. He stoops to collect the floating documents, a motion somber with the weight of undesire.

Douglass, suddenly feeling the effects of drink, improvises an awkward jig. "Cheer up, Lincoln! You are yet the President of these United States!"

Lincoln sucks in his cheeks. "So I am given to understand."

*

After he trounces McClellan in the election of 1864, rumors begin to circulate around the capital of a plot to depose Lincoln and appoint a dictator. The president, suffering an intense bout of melancholia, refuses to see members of his cabinet.

"If anyone can do better than me, let him try his hand," he writes, in a note to congressional leaders. "You boys at the other end of the avenue seem to feel my job is sorely desired. Listen: I am but one man in this ruinous union, which has become nothing but a white elephant, impossible to steer or manage."

*

"And why sugar, Lincoln?"

"The effects of the elixir reach the brain faster."

"It is not just a matter of taste?"

"Certainly not."

"Have you no cause to savor your drink?"

"Of cause I have no end, Douglass. Time—that is the matter."

"Grant makes time."

"He is a soldier. That is his brand."

"And us?"

"We are lovers, Douglass."

*

Douglass finds Lincoln in his study. The lines along his mouth are sunk deep as runnels. "The speech didn't scour. It was a flat failure. The people are disappointed."

"I thought it a fine speech."

"Everett, Seward, and Lamon all thought it bad. I have blundered, Douglass, and made an enemy of brevity."

"It was succinct."

"No, no, Douglass. You are too kind to me. It was a failure. A perfect failure."

*

"Do you, in those moments alone, look into the eyes of your wife?"

"That much depends, Lincoln, on whether I am in a position to do so."

Lincoln offers a throaty laugh. His long earlobes, mossed with fine hairs, jiggle. "I see." He plucks at Douglass's silk cravat. "And from whom does this finery derive?"

Douglass displays a band of teeth, fingers the cloth. "This? Hmmmm. Let me see." He tips the flask. "The good widow Winchester, I believe."

"Yes?"

"If memory serves."

"You have had the good fortune of good widows."

"Indeed."

"You have provided them a great comfort, I suppose."

AWAKE!

"So I am given to understand."

*

"I have just had the oddest dream," Lincoln says. "Do you remember the flat-boat, Mary? Did you know me then? I was there, on the river. The air was like jelly, thick and full of fruit. And do you know what was with me? You will never guess."

Mary does not answer. She is occupied with the task of scratching flowers off the bedside wallpaper with a butter knife.

*

"I was made happiest, by jing, at my election as captain of the volunteers in the Blackhawk War."

"You look something like an Indian," Douglass says. "Your cheeks appear chopped at." They are past the Mason-Dixon, floating from St. Louis into Trapville.

"And then my days railsplitting." Lincoln sips at the flask, wipes his mouth with his wrist, and shambles to his feet. With great ceremony, he spits into one palm, then the other, lifts an invisible hammer over his head, and brings it down onto an equally invisible spike. His height is accentuated by a certain unconsummated grace. "I worked with a fellow named Cooper. His arms were like bolts of pig iron. He celebrated every tie with a song. 'The Sword of Bunker Hill.' 'The Lament of the Irish Immigrant.' Do you know that one, Douglass?"

"No."

Lincoln, still hammering, begins to sing in a reedy baritone:
I'm very lonely now, Mary
For the poor make few new friends

*

"Will you join me, Douglass?"

"Not just yet, Mr. President."

"We laid track from New Salem to Red Bend. In the evenings, Ann would rub my shoulders."

"Ann?"

"With liniment."

"Ann whom?"

Lincoln has sweat through his undershirt. His face is lit with a sudden exhaustion. "Perhaps that is what I meant to remember," he says softly. Lincoln gazes at Douglass for a long while. "They shall set us against one another, friend, we men of honest labor, with our women between us. You do understand that, don't you?"

*

Lincoln's first vision occurs in 1860, following his election as President. He is reclining in his chambers at the Springfield courthouse, facing a looking-glass. In this glass he sees two faces at once, both his own. The first is full of a healthful glow. The second reveals a ghostly paleness. He repeats this experiment no fewer than six times. On each occasion, the illusion reappears.

*

The flask is done at dusk. Both men have stripped down to skivvies. "Honest Abe," Douglass says.

"I cannot tell a lie."

Douglass smiles. "Have you ever kept a pet, Honest Abe?"

"As a lad, I trained a jackrabbit to eat from my hand."

"I should have thought a jackass." Douglass strides to the edge of the flatboat and spits. "Sometimes I dream I am kept as a pet. With many merry widows to feed me carrots and meat and bits of books. My cage is made of woven flax and goldenrod."

"That calls to mind a story, Douglass, of the merchant with a half-wit son. It seems the boy required a sip of molasses before he would to bed each night."

"How has this anything to do with a cage?"

Lincoln frowns. "Yes. I see." Quite independently, the pair dissolve into giggles. "Oh my," Lincoln says.

"Yes?"

"I must relieve myself."

Douglass issues a clarion blare through his fingers: "The business of the presidential bladder must be attended to," he announces. "Please clear a path for the presidential indiscretion."

Lincoln lurches toward the edge of the flatboat. He appears, at best, a man stapled together. "The bank," he says, pawing the air.

"So then, must we by needs speak of the presidential bowels?"

"Stop it now, Douglass. Push on toward the bank."

"Yassah!"

The vessel comes to settle in a stand of reeds. Lincoln tumbles into the water and lets out a whoop. He dogpaddles to the shore, his coarse hair washed off his forehead. Douglass notes the odd shape of his skull, as if someone had pinched him about the jaws and sent the remaining bone ballooning up. He has a small man's face, the eyes

113

of an obedient dog. Lincoln straggles to his feet, britches clinging pinkly to his bottom.

"I am a teapot, Douglass," he hollers. "Here is my spout."

*

Douglass finds Lincoln alone, reclining on a settee in the West Wing. His eyes are shut, and the puffed flesh beneath them is the color of cherrywood. Douglass retreats to the doorway.

"Don't run off, Douglass," Lincoln says, though his eyes remain shut. "I was just now thinking of you."

"Were you?"

"Indeed. I dreamt us together. You were very brave, Douglass. You tried to save me." Lincoln touches his beard. "Did you know, friend, that I suffer from patmos, a kinship with the shades?"

Douglass grins. "Do you?"

"For years, I have known I shall suffer a violent end."

"That is nonsense, sir. You are surely protected."

"I am afraid not, Douglass. That is only a belief to ease the moment. God alone can disarm the cloud of its lightning. Do you agree, Douglass?"

Douglass tries to speak, but his throat constricts, as if clenched by a fist.

Lincoln doesn't seem to notice. "For a man to travel to Africa and rob her of her children—that is worse than murder by my hand. Soon, I believe, the people of the South shall be touched by the better angels of our nature. Consider Goethe: 'Nature cannot but do right eternally.' Are we men not a part of nature?"

"Yes," Douglass says. "On earth and in Heaven."

Lincoln opens his eyes and Douglass notes how red they are, like portals of blood. "I am afraid with all my troubles, I shall never get to the place you speak of, friend."

Douglass is halfway returned to New Bedford before he realizes the source of his disquietude: Lincoln seems to have derived a strange succor from his rumination, as if grief were his own dependable ally.

*

What sort of affiliation is this, Douglass wonders, that seeks to undo a natural repulsion? I do not understand Lincoln, nor he me. We are like two polite giants sharing the same bed and pretending not to mind. Perhaps we are friends because we must not be enemies.

Douglass peers through the telescope he has mounted on a small rise behind the White House. Lincoln is at the window behind his desk, gazing out from the dimmed room. His lips are moving, almost imperceptibly. He looks as if he has been there for years.

*

"I am public property now," Lincoln tells his marshals. "Open the curtains at once." They are returning to the capital from Antietam by carriage. "I shall not cower in this absurd darkness at the very moment when my behavior should exhibit the utmost dignity and composure."

"Mr. President—"

"Who should want to harm me? This is nonsense."

"But sir—"

"And what if I should die?" he mutters. "Would any of you be so much worse off?"

The marshals part the curtains. Lincoln stares into the night, his beaked profile cast in bronze by the carriage lantern. For the rest of the trip, as the corpses and shanties tumble past, his marshals puzzle over this odd vehemence; whether it is simple pride, willed naivete, or a variety of reckless self-determination.

*

Lincoln and Douglass lie together, beneath the stars. Without the gas lamps of Washington and New Bedford, the night sky appears far closer.

"Am I so ugly?" Lincoln says.

"I'm afraid so."

"Ape-like? That is what they say, is it not?"

"Only some of them."

"And the others?"

"*Rawboned*," Douglass says ruefully. "Sometimes *goonish*."

"Would you believe that I dreamed to be a stage actor when I was a lad?"

"Or that I dreamed to be a free man?"

"Please," Lincoln murmurs. "Some restraint, Douglass."

*

"Come away from there," Mary says. "What are you looking at? What is it you see in that infernal mirror?"

*

Douglass lies in the crook of Lincoln's arm. From above, where the night clouds puff like whipping cream, their two forms compose a chain link.

AWAKE!

"Tad plays a sort of theater game in his closet," Lincoln says.

"He is your third?"

"Fourth."

"And the others?"

"Eddie died at three. And Willie, Mary's favorite, just last year. Tad will die too, just before his eighteenth birthday. Sometimes, it seems everything I touch dies."

Douglass lays his hand across Lincoln's chest. "I am not dead."

"No. There is that."

＊

"It seems strange how dreams fill the Bible. I cannot say that I believe in them, but I had the other night an episode which has haunted me ever since. Afterwards, I opened the Bible to the twenty-eighth chapter of Genesis, Jacob's wonderful dream. I turned to another page, then another, and at every turn encountered some reference to a dream or vision." Lincoln rubs his eyes. "Saul. Nebuchadnezzar."

He is standing at the window behind his desk, facing away from his wife, who has entered in her elaborate bedclothes.

"Come away from there, Abraham."

Lincoln can see her reflection in the glass, her mouth set in a line.

"Come to bed. You are talking in riddles again."

"Not riddles, dear. Dreams."

"What is the difference?"

Lincoln glances about. The lamps are dimmed, the brownish light best suited to a seance. Stacks of papers rise around him. "Have you noticed how this office has come to resemble a crypt?"

Mary yawns. "If you would simply keep your affairs in order."

＊

Passing into Greenville, Douglass tosses in his bedclothes. His head aches miserably. Night lends the willows on either bank the appearance of hunched croppers. From behind them, a figure drifts forward, an apparition in gray muslin. Husks of corn lay gnarled in his hair. He stops short of the water, hovering, and moans.

A fury, Douglass thinks. I shall ignore him.

"Yes. I've no business with you, nigger. You are just a fat mouth, a chest full of dull powder. I have come for him. He is mine, now."

"Yours?"

"Surely you don't imagine him to be *yours*?"

The fury opens his black mouth and shivers with laughter.

Douglass shakes Lincoln, thinking to secret him to the other bank. "Lincoln. Arise Lincoln."

Lincoln lies perfectly still, swaddled in his blanket. The night smells sticky and wrongly sweet.

"Please Lincoln, arise!"

*

"About ten days ago I retired late, Mary. I was awaiting word from Appomattox. Do you remember the night? I fell into a slumber, standing right here, on this very spot."

"Abraham. Please."

"Soon I began to dream. I felt a death-like stillness about me. Then I heard subdued sobs, as if a number of people were mourning. I wandered downstairs. There, the silence was broken by the same sobbing. I went from room to room; no living person was in sight, but the same sounds of distress met me as I passed along. The rooms were lit and every object familiar to me, but where were all the people?"

"I am leaving—"

"I was puzzled and alarmed. I kept on until I arrived at the East Room, which I entered. Before me was a catafalque, on which rested a corpse wrapped in funeral vestments."

"Stop this! I will not hear another word."

Lincoln hears her footsteps retreating.

"Around this corpse were stationed soldiers acting as guards and a throng of people gazing upon the corpse, whose face was covered. Others wept pitifully. 'Who is dead in the White House?' I demanded of one of the soldiers. 'The President' was his answer. 'He was killed by an assassin!' Then came a loud burst of grief from the crowd, which woke me from my dream."

He is still at the window, regarding the night. "Well, it is only a dream, Mary. Let us say no more about it, and try to forget it."

Douglass, perched behind a telescope on his hillside, watches Lincoln's lips, at last, grow still.

*

The flatboat glides along toward the Gulf of Mexico. On the far bank, a group of Negroes circles a modest grave. A preacher, his robe frayed and torn, shovels dirt into the pit. A woman cries out. The dawn has made everything wet.

AWAKE!

Lincoln climbs groggily to his feet. "My God," he says. "My head feels like a rifle tamped to fire." He rubs his temples and surveys the scene. "Who are they mourning, Douglass?"

Douglass shakes his head.

"Speak man."

"I don't know."

"Perhaps we can offer a prayer." Lincoln directs the flatboat toward the shore.

"It is too late, sir."

"Have you no compassion, Douglass? Stay a minute and offer condolences. Perhaps the slain—"

"Please, Lincoln, let us pass along."

"They are mourning, friend. We shall exhibit some grace. We must not deaden ourselves to grace."

The preacher pats a final scoop of dirt. The mourners turn, begin to file away from the bier. With a start, Douglass notes a single white face among them: the President's wife, in a plain silk kerchief. Lincoln seems to notice nothing. He presses condolences onto the preacher, whose eyes bug in astonishment.

Returning to the boat, Lincoln draws a breath and slowly exhales. He sets his hand on Douglass's shoulder, steadies himself against a fainting spell. "I am reminded here of a story—"

"Damn you, Lincoln! It is all story with you. Do you not see what is happening?" Douglass shrugs the hand away. He has begun to weep.

Lincoln gazes at the gray morning and lowers himself to a sitting position. His legs dangle, so that his feet are dragged along in the water. To Douglass, they look like a pair of fish struggling exquisitely against the current.

"We are not far from New Orleans," Lincoln says. "We are close now."

*

"There once was a man who found no happiness in his life. He was sad every moment of the day. His duties were many and without mercy. Senators ran to him in anger. Common men blackened their hearts on his behalf. A nation of mothers cursed his name. He hoped to make himself content through an adherence to God's will, but when he examined his beliefs found he held none. His wife went insane, Douglass. His children died like flies. His one love perished." Lincoln's voice deepens and curls, assumes the timbre of dream. "He behaved nobly, but for reasons he could not fathom. His faults were but the shadows his virtues cast. He saw

118

himself grimly advancing on history, but came to understand it was the other way around. He grew bored of his own stories and savored none of his achievements. His single respite was sleep. And then that left him too. Hold me, Douglass. All the strange checkered past seems to crowd now upon my mind."

*

"Do you hear me, Mary? I am speaking of a strange dream."

"Damn your dreams. Dress yourself properly. I shan't be made the object of ridicule in a full theater."

*

"You will understand," Lincoln says. "You are the one man among all of them who must, by needs, understand." He stares at Douglass and Douglass stares back. Each man can hear the other's breath. They are so close they might embrace.

Instead, Lincoln takes up his longpole and pushes off from the bank. Douglass stands on the shore, watching, until the figure is but a gangly figment, dead to duty, dead to memoranda, dead to the human struggle and to the wickedness of blood, alive only to himself and the green of the gulf.

*

On his own deathbed, thirty years later, Douglass will consider a singular vision of Lincoln, his long body laid along the flatboat, his legs dangling, feet cutting through the glassy water, the water washing his glassy feet, the flatboat floating through a city still asleep, floating wakelessly.

WEDNESDAY

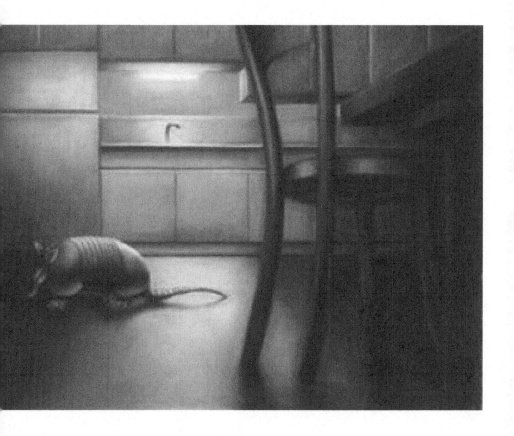

Appliance Song

SHAKESPEARE'S INSOMNIA AND THE CAUSES THEREOF

Franklin H. Head

I.

Insomnia, the lack of "tired Nature's sweet restorer," is rapidly becoming the chronic terror of all men of active life who have passed the age of thirty-five or forty years. In early life, while yet he "wears the rose of youth upon him," man rarely, except in sickness, knows the want of sound, undreaming sleep. But as early manhood is left behind and the cares and perplexities of life weigh upon him, making far more needful than ever the rest which comes only through unbroken sleep, this remedial agent cannot longer be wooed and won. Youth would "fain encounter darkness as a bride and hug it in his arms." To those of riper years the "blanket of the dark" often ushers in a season of terrors—a time of fitful snatches of broken sleep and of tormenting dreams; of long stretches of wakefulness; of hours when all things perplexing and troublesome in one's affairs march before him in sombre procession: in endless disorder, in labyrinths of confusion, in countless new phases of disagreeableness; and at length the morning summons him to labor, far more racked and weary than when he sought repose.

It has been of late years much the fashion in the literature of this subject to attribute sleeplessness to the rapid growth of facilities for activities of every kind. The practical annihilation of time and space by our telegraphs and railroads, the compressing thereby of the labors of months into hours or even minutes, the terrific competition in all kinds of business thereby made possible and inevitable, the intense mental activity engendered in the mad race for fame or wealth, where the nervous and mental force of man is measured against steam and lightning—these are usually credited with having developed what is considered a modern and even an almost distinctively American disease.

As the maxim, "There is nothing new under the sun," is of general application, it may be of interest to investigate if an exception occurs in the case of sleeplessness; if it be true that among our ancestors, before the days of working steam and

123

electricity, the glorious sleep of youth was prolonged through all one's three or four score years.

Medical books and literature throw no light upon this subject three hundred years ago. We must therefore turn to Shakespeare—human nature's universal solvent—for light on this as we would on any other question of his time. Was he troubled with insomnia, then, is the first problem to be solved.

Dr. Holmes, our genial and many-sided poet-laureate, who is also a philosopher, in his *Life of Emerson*, has finely worked out the theory that no man writes other than his own experience: that consciously or otherwise an author describes himself in the characters he draws; that when he loves the character he delineates, it is in some measure his own, or at least one of which he feels its tendencies and possibilities belong to himself. Emerson, too, says of Shakespeare, that all his poetry was first experience.

When we seek to analyze what we mean by the term Shakespeare, to endeavor to define wherein he was distinct from all others and easily pre-eminent, to know why to us he ever grows wiser as we grow wise, we find that his especial characteristic was an unequalled power of observation and an ability accurately to chronicle his impressions. He was the only man ever born who lived and wrote absolutely without bias or prejudice. Emerson says of him that "he reported all things with impartiality; that he tells the great greatly, the small subordinately—he is strong as Nature is strong, who lifts the land into mountain slopes without effort, and by the same rule as she floats a bubble in the air, and likes as well to do the one as the other." Says he, further: "Give a man of talents a story to tell, and his partiality will presently appear: he has certain opinions which he disposes other things to bring into prominence; he crams this part and starves the other part, consulting not the fitness of the thing but his fitness and strength." But Shakespeare has no peculiarity; all is duly given.

Thus it is that his dramas are the book of human life. He was an accurate observer of Nature: he notes the markings of the violet and the daisy; the haunts of the honeysuckle, the mistletoe, and the woodbine. He marks the fealty of the marigold to its god the sun, and even touches the freaks of fashion, condemning in some woman of his time a usage, long obsolete, in accordance with which she adorned her head with "the golden tresses of the dead." But it was as an observer and a delineator of man in all his moods that he was the bright, consummate flower of humanity. His experiences were wide and varied. He had absorbed into himself and made his own the pith and wisdom of his day. As the fittest survives, each age embodies in itself all worthy of preservation in the ages gone before. In Shakespeare's pages we find a reflection, perfect and absolute, of the age of Elizabeth, and therefore of all not transient in the foregone times—of all which is fixed and permanent in our own. He "held the mirror up to Nature." So "his eternal summer shall not fade," because

"He sang of the earth as it will be
When the years have passed away."

If, therefore, insomnia had prevailed in or before his time, in his pages shall we find it duly set forth. If he had suffered, if the "fringed curtains of his eyes were all the night undrawn," we shall find his dreary experiences—his hours of pathetic misery, his nights of desolation—voiced by the tongues of his men and women.

Shakespeare speaks often of the time in life when men have left behind them the dreamless sleep of youth. Friar Laurence says:—

"Care keeps his watch in every old man's eye,
And where care lodges, sleep can never lie;
But where unbruisèd youth with unstuffed brain
Doth couch his limbs, there golden sleep doth reign."

Shakespeare describes, too, with lifelike fidelity, the causes of insomnia, which are not weariness or physical pain, but undue mental anxiety. He constantly contrasts the troubled sleep of those burdened with anxieties and cares, with the happy lot of the laborer whose physical weariness insures him a tranquil night's repose. Henry VI says:—

"And to conclude, the shepherd's homely curds,
His cold thin drink out of his leather bottle,
His wonted sleep under a fresh tree's shade,
All which secure and sweetly he enjoys,
Are far beyond a prince's delicates."

AWAKE!

And Henry V says:—

"'Tis not the balm, the sceptre and the ball,
The sword, the mace, the crown imperial,
The intertissued robe of gold and pearl,
The farcèd title running 'fore the king,
The throne he sits on, nor the tide of pomp
That beats upon the high shore of this world,—
No, not all these, thrice gorgeous ceremony,
Not all these, laid in bed majestical,
Can sleep so soundly as the wretched slave,
Who, with a body filled and vacant mind,
Gets him to rest, crammed with distressful bread;
Never sees horrid night, that child of hell,
But, like a lackey, from the rise to set,
Sweats in the eye of Phoebus, and all night
Sleeps in Elysium . . .
And, but for ceremony, such a wretch,
Winding up days with toil and nights with sleep,
Hath the forehand and vantage of a king."

Prince Henry says, in *Henry IV*:—

"O polished perturbation! Golden care!
That keep'st the ports of slumber open wide
To many a watchful night, sleep with it now!
Yet not so sound and half so deeply sweet
As he whose brow with homely biggin bound
Snores out the watch of night."

In this same play, too, is found the familiar and marvelous soliloquy of Henry IV:—

"How many thousand of my poorest subjects
Are at this hour asleep! O Sleep, O gentle Sleep,
Nature's soft nurse, how have I frighted thee,

That thou no more wilt weigh my eyelids down
And steep my senses in forgetfulness?
Why rather, Sleep, liest thou in smoky cribs,
Upon uneasy pallets stretching thee,
And hushed with buzzing night-flies to thy slumber,
Than in the perfumed chambers of the great,
Under the canopies of costly state,
And lulled with sounds of sweetest melody?
O thou dull god, why liest thou with the vile
In loathsome beds, and leav'st the kingly couch
A watch-case, or a common 'larum-bell?
Wilt thou upon the high and giddy mast
Seal up the ship-boy's eyes, and rock his brains
In cradle of the rude, imperious surge,
And in the visitation of the winds,
Who take the ruffian billows by the top,
Curling their monstrous heads, and hanging them
With deafening clamor in the slippery shrouds,
That with the hurly, death itself awakes?
Canst thou, O partial Sleep, give thy repose
To the wet sea-boy in an hour so rude,
And in the calmest and most stillest night,
With all appliances and means to boot,
Deny it to a king? Then, happy low, lie down!
Uneasy lies the head that wears a crown."

Caesar, whom Shakespeare characterizes as "the foremost man of all this world," says:—

"Let me have men about me that are fat;
Sleek-headed men, and such as sleep o' nights."

And again, it is not an "old man broken with the storms of state" whom he describes when he says:—

AWAKE!

> "Thou hast no figures nor no fantasies
> Which busy care draws in the brains of men;
> Therefore thou sleep'st so sound."

The poet also in various passages expresses his emphatic belief as to what is the brightest blessing or the deadliest calamity which can be laid upon our frail humanity. Rarely is a blessing invoked which does not include the wish for tranquil sleep; and this, too, as the best and greatest boon of all. His gracious benediction may compass honors and wealth and happiness and fame—that one's "name may dwell forever in the mouths of men;" but

> "The earth hath bubbles as the water hath,
> And these are of them."

as compared with the royal benison, "Sleep give thee all his rest."

The spectres of the princes and Queen Anne, in *Richard III*, invoking every good upon Richmond, say:—

> "Sleep, Richmond, sleep in peace and wake in joy."

And again:—

> "Thou quiet soul, sleep thou a quiet sleep."

Romeo's dearest wish to Juliet is:—

> "Sleep dwell upon thine eyes; peace in thy breast."

The crowning promise of Lady Mortimer, in *Henry IV*, is that:—

> "She will sing the song that pleaseth thee,
> And on thy eyelids crown the god of sleep."

Titania promises her fantastic lover:—

"I'll give thee fairies to attend on thee,
And they shall fetch thee jewels from the deep,
And sing, while thou on pressèd flowers dost sleep."

Titus, welcoming again to Rome the victorious legions, says of the heroes who have fallen:—

"There greet in silence, as the dead are wont,
And sleep in peace, slain in your country's wars,"

promising them that in the land of the blest

"are no storms,
No noise, but silence and eternal sleep."

Constantly also in anathemas throughout the plays are invoked, as the deadliest of curses, broken rest and its usual accompaniment of troublous dreams. Thus note the climax in Queen Margaret's curse upon the traitorous Gloucester:—

"If Heaven have any grievous plague in store
Exceeding those that I can wish upon thee,
Oh, let them keep it till thy sins be ripe,
And then hurl down their indignation
On thee, the troubler of the poor world's peace!
The worm of conscience still begnaw thy soul!
Thy friends suspect for traitors while thou liv'st,
And take deep traitors for thy dearest friends!
No sleep close up that deadly eye of thine,
Unless it be while some tormenting dream
Affrights thee with a hell of ugly devils!"

The witch, in *Macbeth*, cataloguing the calamities in store for the ambitious Thane, says:—

AWAKE!

> "Sleep shall neither night nor day
> Hang upon his pent-house lid;
> He shall live a man forbid."

It is curious also to remark, in the various lists of griefs which make life a burden and a sorrow, how often the climax of these woes is the lack of sleep, or the troubled dreams bearing their train of "gorgons, hydras, and chimeras dire," which come with broken rest. Lady Percy says to Hotspur:—

> "Why hast thou lost the fresh blood in thy cheeks,
> And given my treasures and my rights of thee
> To thick-eyed musing and curst melancholy?
> Tell me, sweet lord, what is't that takes from thee
> Thy stomach, pleasure, and thy golden sleep?"

Macbeth says:—

> "But let the frame of things disjoint, both the worlds suffer,
> Ere we will eat our meal in fear, and sleep
> In the affliction of these terrible dreams
> That shake us nightly; better be with the dead."

In *Othello* is a striking picture of the sudden change, in the direction we are considering, which comes over a tranquil mind from the commission of a great crime. Iago says to Othello, after he has wrought "the deed without a name":—

> "Not poppy nor mandragora,
> Nor all the drowsy syrups of the world,
> Shall ever medicine thee to that sweet sleep
> Which thou own'dst yesterday."

The greatest punishment which comes to Macbeth after the murder of Duncan is lack of sleep. Nowhere in the language, in the same space, can be found so many pictures of the blessedness of repose as in the familiar lines:—

"Methought I heard a voice cry, 'Sleep no more!
Macbeth does murder sleep,' the innocent sleep;
Sleep that knits up the ravelled sleave of care,
The death of each day's life, sore labor's bath,
Balm of hurt minds, great Nature's second course,
Chief nourisher in life's feast."

And the principal reason which deters Hamlet from suicide is the fear that even if he does sleep well "after life's fitful fever is over," still, that sleep may be full of troubled dreams.

"To sleep, perchance to dream. Ay, there's the rub;
For in that sleep of death what dreams may come
When we have shuffled off this mortal coil,
Must give us pause."

Richard III says, when the catalogue of his crimes is full, and when he "sees as in a map the end of all":—

"The sons of Edward sleep in Abraham's bosom,
And Anne, my queen, hath bid the world good night."

In addition to the fuller phrases wherein are shown the blessedness of sleep, or the remediless nature of its loss, many brief sentences occur scattered throughout the plays, and emphasizing the same great lesson. For instance:—

"Now o'er one half the world
Nature seems dead, and wicked dreams abuse
The curtained sleep."

"With Him above
To ratify our work, we may again
Give to our tables meat, sleep to our nights."

"You lack the season of all natures, sleep."

AWAKE!

"My soul is heavy, and I fain would sleep."

"For never yet one hour in his bed
Have I enjoyed the golden dew of sleep."

"For some must watch and some must sleep,
So runs the world away."

"How sweet the moonlight sleeps upon that bank."

"The best of rest is sleep."

"Our little lives are rounded with a sleep."

The various passages cited above prove and illustrate that no author has written so feelingly, so appreciatingly, as Shakespeare on the subject of sleep and its loss.

The diligent commentators on his works have investigated laboriously the sources from which he drew his plots and many of the very lines of his poems. He was a great borrower; absorbing, digesting, and making his own much of the material of his predecessors. But it is a noteworthy fact, that none of the exquisite lines in praise of sleep—that gift which the Psalmist says the Lord giveth to his beloved—can be traced to other source than the master. These are jewels of his own; transcripts from his own mournful experience. In middle life he remembered hopelessly the tranquil sleep of his lost youth, as

"He that is stricken blind cannot forget
The precious treasure of his eyesight lost."

He had suffered from insomnia, and he writes of this, not "as imagination bodies forth the forms of things *unknown*," but as one who, in words burning with indestructible life, lays open to us the sombre record of what was experience before it was song; who makes us the sharers of his griefs; who would awaken in the similarly afflicted of all time that compassionate sympathy which goes out to those whose burdens are almost greater than they can bear.

FROM THE INSOMNIA DRAWINGS
LOUISE BOURGEOIS

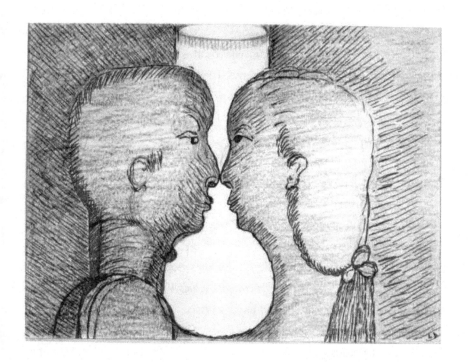

The Insomnia Drawings (detail), 1994-1995
220 mixed media works on paper of varying dimensions
Daros Collection, courtesy Cheim & Read, New York
Photo: Christopher Burke

NEVER SLEEP AGAIN
GWENDA BOND

No one in my fifth grade class slept for fear of bloody death. Well, that's not precisely true—Kathy and Jodi and Bridget with one T, I'm sure they slept fine. I barely remember their place in the social order.

My classmates who didn't sleep were the people whose opinions I sought on important issues: Was I fat? Wasn't my older brother's friend Scott cute? Were candy pink Reeboks in or out? They mattered. They stayed awake. I never considered myself the *est* of the cool kids, but it was my own fault. I hadn't seen A *Nightmare on Elm Street.*

"Tell me about the boyfriend's death scene," I begged Chris, who became a doctor when he grew up. I had a crush on him. Chris blinked, said, "They're supposed to talk on the phone, phone sex, but wuss goes to sleep instead and—"

Bridgett cut him off. "God, you suck. You always tell the blood spatter wrong," she said. Acid in her voice and hate in her heart.

Bridgett with two Ts was our real expert. She was also a bitch goddess, the Alexis Carrington of our school. Bridgett's parents would let her watch anything.

"Nancy's boyfriend, right? She knows he's being killed," Bridgett said, smacking Hubba Bubba gum. "She's trying and trying to call him. But he's out. ZZZZZZZZZ. Freddy sucks him into the sheets—a place where Nancy has never been and she's sad about that. Because this is no wuss, this is *Johnny Depp*, and she's totally not hot enough for him to begin with . . ."

Bridgett had perfected a description of what happened with the boyfriend's blood. Her most memorable summer vacation had been to Yellowstone.

"It's just like Old Faithful," she said. "Shooting up in a geyser onto the ceiling, gushing like a backward waterfall. More blood than Johnny Depp even had. It's the blood of all *his* victims." She paused for dramatic effect: "Freddy's victims."

I shuddered at his name. We all did.

*

Consider: when you sleep, a madman attacks you. Not just any madman either, but a sexual predator, a child molester. In your dreams, you are powerless as a child and he can take your life from you any way he wants. You won't ever wake up. The only defense is to not sleep.

The details were simple, but sexy. Take the parents. Can you imagine your parents as part of an angry mob, murdering someone and getting away with it? My parents were principals. The movie parents were starring in evil's own personal soap opera. Never mind that the teenage characters had sex and talked about it. Or that Nancy was afraid she was going crazy. Freddy Krueger had those long, long knife fingers. That filthy red and green sweater. The soundtrack, all sing-song chanting in creepy child voice stereo. But I always came back around to the parents. The mother put thick metal bars on the windows, preventing her daughter's escape. Once a murderer, always one . . .

Bridgett held us rapt for entire lunch periods and break times, on late night three-way phone calls. She was particularly insightful about Nancy's mother. What with the addiction, depression, and estrangement from Nancy's father, she couldn't have been that far outside Bridgett's own experience. Her dark family life gave her the ability to speak with authority, to be our queen.

Chris did have one major thing over Bridgett though, besides being cuter. Even if he couldn't recount it for shit, he'd seen the most recent Freddy movie, *Dream Warriors*. He said the movie made it clear that doubt would get us killed. This was all true and happening and we really shouldn't risk sleep. In this one, Nancy died.

Like most horror movies, these were better as urban legends, relayed by one person to another. The more we talked about them, the scarier they were. We shared No Doz tablets and cans of Jolt Cola swiped from older siblings.

Somehow, no one in our class had heard about my history of sleeplessness. For most kids, the dark gets scary when they're young and innocent, then they grow out of it. My hysterical insomnia hit when I was about eight, a couple of years before I got interested in movies about nightmares.

*

I kept on every lamp in my room at night—two Strawberry Shortcakes and a hideous antique. Each night, all night, I read. I slept for a few hours after the sun came up.

AWAKE!

If there was a noise outside during the night, I stopped reading and listened hard until it stopped. I was half-convinced that my salt-and-pepper mutt Trixie took on the forces of evil and chaos in our yard. Trixie and the spiny tree outside my window were the only things keeping me safe. My dad had planted the tree in front of my window the day I was born. Maybe all parents *do* want to keep their children captive.

My parents finally figured out I wasn't sleeping. They tried to force me.

I had to drag my camouflage sleeping bag into their bedroom, where I could be monitored, and sleep on the floor. In the dark. It turned out sleep was good. I liked sleep. A week later when they tried to force me back into my own room, I said no. Screamed no, cried and yelled it. My older brother came out and yelled some back, disgusted by my weakness and tears. Eventually I was allowed to climb back into the sleeping bag.

My dad was principal of our school, but it was divided into two separate buildings. Grades four through eight were held in a giant gothic fortress on a hill overlooking our tiny downtown, while kindergarten through fourth took place in a more traditional building a few miles away.

The year of my insomnia, I'd taken the bus up to the hill every day after school to meet my dad and brother so we could ride home together. The older girls in my brother's class wrote salacious notes in the back of his yearbooks. They treated me like a pet. They loved to braid my hair after school or take me out to the swings with them, where we kicked our legs out over a kudzu-covered cliff.

When I came through the door the day after my middle of the night fit, the PA started right away. I knew instantly what was happening. My brother had a large tape deck at home. He'd recorded the whole thing. Now he was playing it for his school.

"No! No! Don't make me go in there! Don't make me! It'll be dark! No!" I sobbed, screamed, raged.

"Honey, it's okay. Nothing's going to happen to you." My mom, pleading.

"Calm down! Behave yourself!" My dad, doing his best authoritarian.

"She just wants attention, she's crazy! What's wrong with you? Just go to sleep!" My brother.

I screeched.

My dad got to the PA as soon as he could and cut it off. No doubt he paddled my brother, because you could still do that then. He *deserved* it.

136

I stood in the hallway, mortified, until someone left the administrative office and spotted me. It was one of the older girls.

"You okay?" she asked.

I had to lie.

"He paid me to throw a fit," I said. "He paid me five dollars. He never said anything about taping me. It was a set up."

She looked at me, unsure how to react. A few other girls joined us.

I laughed. "He got me," I said.

My brother came out into the hallway then, face still red from his encounter with dad.

"I hate you," I said. "I would *never* have done it if I knew you were going to pretend that it was *real*. You are the world's biggest jerk, with your stupid pink Don Johnson T-shirts!" I wanted to cry. I laughed again, "You got me. Jerk."

He stayed quiet. He let me say it all.

They didn't believe me, those sharp-tongued, long-haired girls. They were kind enough to not speak to my brother for the rest of the day anyway, to take me out to the swings, to never mention it again.

If we'd gone to school in the same building, everyone would have known. I would have had to migrate to Indonesia or transfer to the private school in the mountains for juvenile delinquents. As it was, I mostly escaped. Oh, I'd get the occasional pitying glance from a teacher who'd heard the tape, but no one in my family ever said anything to me about leaving the lights on again.

*

Sleep was an easy scare. Anything could happen while you were sleeping. Bridgett had told me about a death scene in another movie she'd seen with a lead character called Jason. Jason impaled someone on a sword while they were in bed, stabbing up through the mattress. After that, I checked under my bed before climbing into it, every time.

The only real fallout from the recording episode was that my parents forbid me from seeing scary movies. That was okay though, because not only did Bridgett's parents not care what she watched, they didn't care what her friends saw either.

We planned a sleepover. Our friend Nikki and I would stay over at Bridgett's trailer that Friday. We felt like we were in a movie, scheming something grand, and not a tiny trespass on the rules. I felt a little weird about spending the night in a trailer. They were always blowing apart in tornadoes on the news.

Bridgett's mom drove us to the video rental place in her cramped blue Chevette. The sheet metal building housed a one room selection that was terrible on every score except horror and porn. We rented the first two *Nightmares*, then waited for Bridgett's parents to go to sleep

"One, two, Freddy's coming for you . . ." The song lived up to our playground renderings. *"Three, four, better lock your door . . . Five, six, grab a crucifix . . ."* Two girls jumped rope in sunshine while they sang, the brightness infusing the scene with a genuine creepiness.

Bridgett's TV was tiny, so we huddled together in front of it. Nancy's friend Tina was brutally killed. Nancy's hair turned gray overnight. All these familiar things played out, but they didn't feel right. They weren't exactly how I'd imagined them. Sometimes they were thin; sometimes things just didn't translate on the screen.

Having seen the movie a dozen times, Bridgett couldn't stop herself from narrating key scenes. "Here comes Old Faithful!"

While her boyfriend, Johnny Depp, is being killed, Nancy unplugs her phone. It rings anyway. She answers and Freddy tells her he's her boyfriend now. His tongue snakes from the bottom of the receiver, which has morphed into his burnt-flesh face.

I was horrified. That had *sounded* scary, but it just looked like the acne-marred faces of the boys at school. Worse, Freddy resembled a campy transvestite in the closing sequence, chasing Nancy through her nest of booby traps and trip wires.

I hadn't slept more than an hour or two a night in months: for this? How could Nancy really believe she was going crazy? *People died.* You couldn't crazy people into dying. I wanted to yell at her to stop being so whiny. To think.

The sequel was abysmal.

Bridgett sat up after we finished watching the movies. "Let's go over the rules," she said.

We had rehashed it all so often.

"Don't sleep, don't say his name, don't dream," she solemnly recited.

Nikki said nothing. She'd seen it before.

"What did you think?" Bridgett asked, annoyed at my lack of interest.

"The scene with the swimming pool in *Freddy's Revenge* is *stupid*," I said.

Nikki seemed impressed by this analysis.

Bridgett drew back and looked at me. "Well, yeah," she said. "But what about Tina in the body bag . . ."

I was bored. I went to sleep.

They put my light pink training bra in the freezer while I was out. Things went back to something resembling normal. We stopped talking about killer dreams and popping caffeine pills.

Bridgett died of a meth overdose in her mid-twenties. My brother became a youth minister. And I sleep every night in the dark.

EMERALDS WOULD BE INVISIBLE WHERE YOU ARE

Dara Wier

Now it is green in this darkness persisting & sudden
And so it is there are no shadows for us to look into, it is
All as if everything that is happening is happening so far
Away from us we are unable to approach it, we are unable
Without you to direct us, we have no means at this time
Toward on the way to where we would go were we able,
Were our wherewithal enabled with triggers of you to
Provide us with all that we should have to be near you
With green, to be near you with thunderings ultra announce-
Ments with aftermaths in ever-widening circles of you
Are a bit of rock dropped into an undisturbed ocean, you
Are waves of telltale and hearsay and vagrant whispers,
You are a staircase a ladder a rope in the middle of nowhere
And we woefully are elsewhere are we greenly beginning.

AND SO THEY SLEEP
CLARO
(TRANSLATION BY BRIAN EVENSON)

Before my encounter with Pranx, inanimate objects were for me only stub-born stones which a blow from thought's hammer, applied at the right moment, pulverized without there ever—ever!—ringing out the slightest echo. Matter, in its lethargic, congealed, mute form is at best a pedestal onto which we lift the mounted fragments of our illusions, but at least this pedestal is solid, without eyes and without memory, incapable of contradiction or cunning; soft flows of sentimental cream and avalanches of candied ideas hardly matter to it. The table upon which I rested my elbows had retained of its woodworker—or more likely from workers working in some anonymous sawmill—neither his doubts nor his fears, but was the rectangular denial of all the secret eddies which, most certainly, plagued the psyche of its creator. Already dead, the table wasn't burdened with a desire for immortality. I would have liked to give back to the earth at four equidistant points the invisible thrust that it inflicted upon my thwarted mass.

So I lived alone, surrounded by innumerable objects whose very essence was situated mid-way between a usefulness that I neglected and a history that I didn't know—they were objects deprived of deliberate beauty, serving a cause for which I had no special affinity. Neither witnesses nor servants, they perfectly peopled the void of my existence. I say "the void," but this is less to lament some personal failure than to designate geometrically the non-encumbered space that I had preserved with the passing of the years.

Then Pranx came and I bit my tongue, unless it was the other way around.

*

The truth demands that I clarify that it was I who had summoned Pranx. I want-ed to get rid of my books, all of my books, which I'd ended up judging too noisy, too rowdy. While sustaining one another quasi-religiously on the shelves, they conducted between them, I very much felt, a mute war, and the memories I retained of some of their pages emitted, coming up against one another, a disagreeable sound, sandpaper on a fresh wound, coarse laughter choked off by drinking straight from the bottle; in short, my books were expressing themselves without my knowledge, and I saw coming the moment when they would end up giving off the odor of rotten eggs. So I decided to get rid of them.

Pranx was a sort of junk dealer whom I had come across many times in a café where I went, once or twice a week, seduced by the immense amnesiac lump which the counter represented in my eyes, the counter whose scratched wood and worn zinc was like the abscissa and ordinate of an imperceptible curve that could never disturb the eructations of the clients grafted onto it. I liked this contrast and, in my slightly caffeine-stained silence, I felt myself an accomplice of the wood, the zinc, a neat line in my own turn.

But I wasn't deaf and I had ended up understanding that Pranx bought and sold books, emptied attics and libraries, and this without moodiness, the opposite of his colleagues who couldn't stop from titillating some naïve clitoridian secret tucked away at the back of the snatch of these dusty works which, it went without saying, replaced a long-gone wife. Their libidinal approach to books had always disgusted me, and I was grateful to this Pranx for being the indifferent pimp of their destiny.

I approached him one morning as he was putting his cap back on and was preparing to push open the door of the café. Taking advantage of the ambient hubbub, like a snake slipping through loquacious foliage, I slid a few words his way concerning my problem, then offered him my card and we arranged to meet the following week.

*

I should have killed him. I should have brought the base of the living room lamp down on the nape of his neck, or driven the butcher's knife lying around on my kitchen counter into his stomach fat. I should have kissed him on the mouth to stun him then garroted him with one of my shoelaces. I should have sunk my fingers into his eyes while crushing his balls in my fist. I should never have opened the door for him, never open, never, ever—but it is too late, the Pranx virus has spread, I am henceforth "pranxed," permanently, and I doubt there exists somewhere in this world an anti-Pranx capable of freeing me from the nightmare which is, today, mine, a nightmare that I wish on my worst enemy: Pranx.

*

Barely having entered, Pranx went to sit on my sofa, more precisely in the middle of the sofa, placing on either side of his thighs, flattened out, two hands with fingers that were, to my taste, a little too long. The last phalanx of his two pinkies was missing, but above all it was the ring on his right hand you noticed, an enormous ring mounted with a sort of sea monster whose tentacles ran over to the two neighboring fingers. He immediately felt my gaze on this absolutely tasteless jewel and thought it best to append a commentary.

It's my conscience, said he.

As I didn't reply, he burst out laughing. It was starting to rain and for a brief moment I had the impression that the raindrops passed through me like x-rays, exposing my dripping skeleton.

How long do you need to assess the sum total of my books and when do you think you can get rid of them?

It's not that simple, he said.

What do you mean?

I didn't know you had so many.

And yet I told you the other day at the café that there were . . .

I'm not talking about books. But about all this.

All what?

He rose and slowly walked around the living room, from time to time placing his index finger on the objects piled up a little everywhere, on bookshelves, tables, radiators, in the smallest corners of the room. He even moved forward into the hallway, where they were perhaps most numerous, and if I hadn't called out he would without any doubt have crossed the threshold of my bedroom.

How are they bothering you?

At the time, my question seemed to me incongruous, as if I had been expecting a sugary taste but a vilely bitter flavor had settled onto my tongue.

He came back in his tracks and went to stand in front of the window. I saw him bend forward slightly until his forehead touched the windowpane—and I felt in my mouth the coolness that his skin must have experienced at that precise instant.

AWAKE!

His shoulders lifted, but just one notch, as if there existed between his shoulder blades a machinery subject to sudden breakdowns. It couldn't have been a sob. Nor a sign of contempt. Pranx was a sick man. And I wished to stay healthy as long as possible.

*

Then he spoke, in a tired voice, like a narrator who knows himself doomed to some monstrous parade, and who is already floating in the ether of a filthy jar.

All these objects, he droned, all these things that you have pilled together . . . They're suffering, they're exhausted, hours go by and they don't have any respite. Can't you feel how of the sleep of being used or of admired is withheld from them? Take that glove, over there, that leather glove lying on that walking stick, it's waiting for a hand, and somewhere a hand waits for it, a hand which would slip into it shuddering with pleasure, its leather is strained by expectancy to the limit, it writhes though motionless, believe me, it writhes, it is twisted up deep within its motionlessness.

He picked it up and pressed it against his lips, then closed his eyes.

Objects need sleep, the sleep of objects; yours are like amputated hands, severed feet, heads torn off of the trunk of life which keep on growing. It's unbearable. It's abominable. I hear them, don't you? The material they are made of doesn't experience the blessed stupor of the worn, the tremendous stupor of the aestheticizing gaze. It's a material given over to itself, to its emptiness, and there is nothing worse for an inanimate object than this forced insomnia, this enslavement of the senses, this withheld night. They will become, if it hasn't happened already, monsters. Look! That lighter whose notched flywheel you never caress: it's a monster! It keeps watch, keeps watch, keeps watch, it's bursting with it, it doesn't even know what a flame is anymore, all the eyes of all its molecules are red and fastened on the white light which you impose on them. What do you think happens to manufactured things when nothing comes to impregnate them?

This last question frightened me so much with its grotesque power that I kicked Pranx out, without brutality but without consideration, and, I must admit, without meeting hardly any resistance on his part.

That was a week ago.

The question of the insomnia of inanimate objects, like the supposed suicide of certain animal species and the eventual attainment of articulate language by primates, is something one can easily return to the bottom drawer of our irritating brain. But sometimes this drawer stays stuck, gaping open, hostile.

After Pranx's departure, I sank into a state of perpetual drowsiness, my gestures aborted themselves, I often tripped, pissed next to the toilet bowl, regularly over-turned my lukewarm coffee on my knees, couldn't even manage to take a shower any more, dreamed intermittently, mumbled, drooled, sleeping often next to the living room rug or at the foot of my bed.

During this time, they didn't sleep. Something along the lines of madness circled in the inorganic cage of their stupefied molecules. Matter bit into itself, almost took pleasure in its own growing hysteria, having too long ago reached beyond the limits of exhaustion. The wood of handles wrapped up in a contempt for a human grip, the iron of blades deprived of the taste of entrails, the ceramic of cups that no lip came to kiss, the glass of light fixtures, the plastic of furnishings, the straw of chairs, the fabric of hangings, everything which formed the disconcerted flesh of my inert possessions was jealous of my now sovereign power to pass away, to relieve my cells of their vain agitation of bygone days, and to know the magnificent unmortaring of consciousness, its slow octopetal fall into the abyss of time.

And this jealousy became revenge. The more they were crushed by their silly impossible death, the more my old me was melting, to the point that within me finally all stray impulse to tame the world through language clouded over and went wrong. From then on, in my rare and imperfect moments of lucidity, I perceived no more than the pranx-soul of things, a sort of raw organism condemned to mime the inanimate without enjoying its delicious comatose state. I was the spineless hostage of an irritated army composed of all possible pranxian insomnias.

To say that this paradox—on one side life reduced to its idiotic drift, on the other the drowsiness prohibited to inert things—triggered an involuntary start in me would be exaggerated.

I left my house, which today Pranx lives in. I think I've understood that he pos-sesses numerous residences in the city, left vacant by people who had called upon his services. I come across him sometimes, in this same café where I spotted him long ago, but neither the counter nor I dare separate to greet him; we remain wisely coupled, encamped in our post-Pranxian retreat, in fear of a cruel awakening which would condemn us to that pendulum movement which is, so it seems, life.

INVISIBLE BOX
BRIAN EVENSON

In retrospect, it was easy for her to see it had been a mistake to have sex with a mime. At the time, though, she had been drunk enough that it seemed like a good idea. Sure, she had been a little surprised, once she had coaxed him upstairs, when he refused to speak, and even more surprised by his refusal to wipe off his face paint or shuck his beret, but, whatever, so what: it would give her a story to tell at parties.

But, ever since, she'd had trouble sleeping. She could manage a fitful hour but then woke up, imagining him there again above her, naked save for his facepaint and beret and white gloves. She watched as, straddling her, he carefully felt out an invisible box around them. He kept making gestures to remind her about the box, feeling it out again, steadying her as she approached one imaginary edge, running his flattened palms along the box's ceiling just before penetrating her. It was a hell of a thing, at once funny and deeply disturbing, and distracting as hell.

When he was coming, pretending to cry out silently, she suddenly realized this was not a story she could bring herself to tell at parties. Half-passed out, she lazily watched him lift the imaginary box off of them, get up and get dressed, then lift the box back in place, over her. She drifted off feeling it there around her, edges softly gleaming, holding her in.

She woke up early the next morning to find herself smeared with white face paint, as well as a few loops of black, like bruises, from his lips. She got up and brewed some coffee, had some toast, vomited. Her head felt wrapped in batting. The mime had not even been good in bed, though he had mimed being good in bed when she had picked him up. No, she thought, he had been more interested in his imaginary box than in her.

So she had slept with a mime, so what? In any case, it was over now, over and done.

*

But it wasn't over, nor was it done. True, she didn't think about the mime for the rest of the day, but later, that night, just as she was lying down to sleep, she felt something. There was the box, rising up around her. She closed her eyes and tried to sleep but kept seeing the box, its edges burning in flashes on the inside of her eyelids. It was hard to sleep feeling it was there, and when she finally did sleep it was fitfully, dreaming of the mime moving inside of her, shoulders hunching to avoid the ceiling of the imaginary box, white face floating like a buoy in the darkness.

She brushed her hand through the box, but it remained undisturbed. She threw back the covers and got a drink and climbed back into bed, beside the box this time, but no, somehow the box was still over her, holding her in. No matter where she went on the bed it was there. *This is ridiculous*, she thought, and tried to sleep, but instead sat there, staring at the inside of the non-existent box, wondering how to get rid of it.

She got up and wandered the apartment, read a little in an armchair, made herself some warm milk, drank it. She began to feel a little sleepy. She nodded in and out in the chair, finally got up and went into the bedroom, climbed back into bed. An instant later she was wide awake, staring again at the inside of the box.

*

Most of the night was like that, with her oppressed by the box that wasn't even there. She slept a little in the chair, on the floor, but never for long, mostly lying in the bed, in the non-existent box, wide awake, feeling absurd. *I should kill that fucking mime*, she thought around four in the morning. A little after five she wondered if there were support groups for women who had slept with mimes. Five minutes later, she started to wonder if the mime had worn a real or an imaginary condom. She kept picturing his exaggerated motions as he put it on. If she had a baby, would it be wearing a beret and white gloves? *Goddamit*, she thought at 5:23 a.m., her eyes puffy, *what's wrong with me?*

She must have fallen asleep for a few minutes anyway, for by the time she awoke light was streaming through the window and the box was gone. Relieved, she called her office and left a message saying she'd be late. She slept a few hours. The rest of the day was a little hazy, her responses slower than normal, and there was a point in the meeting where she completely blanked out, came to herself seconds later to find the client staring at her strangely. She recouped best she could, waded through the rest of the day, left right at five.

*

I'll sleep well tonight, she told herself on the drive home. She collapsed onto the bed before dinner with the last of the sun coming in through the window, fell asleep in her clothes.

She woke up an hour later in the dark, mouth dry, blouse rucked up around her breasts. In the dark she could feel the box there around her. Suddenly she was wide awake. She could not get back to sleep. She wanted to weep. Instead, she lay there feeling the box, trying to ignore it, trying to pretend it wasn't there. *But no,* she thought, *I'm not pretending. It's an imaginary box; it isn't there.* But thinking this didn't seem to help.

*

It was one night among many, each of them shading into each other, each essentially coming down to the same thing: her lying in bed staring through a non-existent box at the ceiling. In the days that followed she tried everything she could think of. She slept naked, she slept clothed, sober, drunk, half-naked, half-clothed, half-sober, half-drunk. She took sleeping pills, which seemed to work for a few hours but didn't make her feel any less tired once she woke up. She changed the sheets; the box was still there. *I should kill that fucking mime,* she thought. She turned the mattress over; the box was still there. She tried to sleep on the couch but even though the box wasn't over her she could feel it in the next room, gently shimmering. She tried to sleep at a friend's house but somehow could still feel the box even from there, blocks away, waiting for her.

She started seeing a psychiatrist who tried to give her *strategies for coping. Maybe,* he suggested after five or six sessions, *you need to give in to your inner mime, so to speak. My inner mime?* she wondered. She listlessly attended two or three more sessions, and then stopped.

Which left her where, exactly? In bed, beneath the box, having difficulty sleeping, eyes redder, mind more and more distracted, wishing every night, as she tried to close her eyes and found they wouldn't close, that she was dead. I'll try anything, she kept telling herself, I'll do anything. Just as long as I can get some sleep.

*

Which is what led her, one night, at three or perhaps twenty past three or perhaps somewhat closer to four—hard to say since there had been so many nights since in which she had done the same thing—to begin thinking with two different parts of her head at once. One part of her head was thinking, as it had thought at least once per night, that she should kill that fucking mime, but the other part was thinking that no, perhaps not kill but fuck him again and this time, after he came, get him to take his fucking box away with him. One part of her head was walking into the kitchen and taking a knife from the block and sliding it into her purse but the other part was thinking what it would say to get the mime to go home with her again, how she would first find him and then fuck him, or no, stab him dead, back and forth until, when she came to herself again and was thinking with only one part of her head, there she was, alone, in the dead of night, in the street, searching for her mime, not knowing whether she would have sex with him or kill him or perhaps both. It was useless, she knew, to look for him so late, but there she was, walking, half-dressed, walking, and now the same thing seemed to happen almost every night, almost without her knowing it, that strange moment where her thinking split into either side of her head and she seemed to fall into the gap between, and by the time she had managed to clamber out, she was out alone on the streets, looking for a mime, only a mime would do.

*

And perhaps it is best to leave her here, half-asleep and wandering, grasping at straws that don't exist, for what good can possibly come of any of this? At best she will soon have butchered a mime in her bed or will end up dead herself. At worst, she will soon find herself enclosed by not just one imaginary box, but by two. That she might actually work her way free, that she might actually, for once, sleep through the night, ever again, seems the least likely possibility of all, even to her. So, let's leave her, let's tuck the covers up around her neck and take a step or two backwards. Let's turn out the light and—despite the soft gleam of her open eyes in the darkness, despite the sounds of her tossing and turning within her box, despite, as night deepens, her little groans of frustration—let's smile and, lying, tell ourselves yes, everything is all right, yes, shhh, yes, she's finally asleep.

THE ORANGE
Simon Armitage

Ricky Wilson couldn't sleep. He got up and went for a walk.
It was 4 o'clock in the morning. There was no one around
except for a drunk sleeping it off in the doorway of Vidal Sassoon.
Then an orange came rolling towards Ricky down Albion Street.
It trundled in his direction before clipping a curbstone and jumping
straight into his hands, like a lost puppy re-united with its owner.
The orange was a little dusty and slightly misshapen from
its journey, but after a quick polish with his cravat and a bit
of molding in his hands, the fruit was restored. He stared
at it under the glow of the streetlamps. It looked very appealing.
Very appealing indeed. In fact Ricky was suddenly seized
with the notion that all his bodily cravings could be satisfied
by the quenching juice and zesty pulp of that ample
citrus fruit sitting in his palm, so without a moment's hesitation
he plunged his thumbnail into the pithy skin and squeezed its
entire contents down his throat. It was then that he heard footsteps.
He thrust the mashed-up orange into his jacket pocket and looked
ahead. A little girl in bare feet came running up to him.
She was wearing a torn, grey pinafore dress and a dirty white
blouse. She couldn't have been more than six or seven, and
was clearly distressed. "Mister, have you seen an orange heading
this way?" "No," lied Ricky, licking the tangy residue from
his lips. Her shoulders dropped. She said, "They say my father
is an illegal immigrant and tomorrow they will deport him
to Albania. I went to Armley prison tonight for one last hug
but they turned me away. I stood outside the prison walls
and shouted his name. Through the bars of his cell he blew
me a final kiss and threw me an orange. But I stumbled on the

sloping streets of this steep city and my orange has disappeared in the night." Obviously she had a heavy Albanian accent, almost unintelligible, in fact, but for the sake of comprehension her remarks are paraphrased here. She fell to her knees and sobbed. Ricky felt like a rotten piece of shit. "What color was it?" he asked. At school, humor would often mitigate his wrong-doings. "I wanted to eat every morsel of that orange, even the skin. Its juice was my father's blood, and the flesh was his spirit," said the girl. "Why don't I help you look for it?" Ricky offered. The little girl looked up at Ricky with a face like a silver coin at the bottom of a deep well caught by the momentary light of a footman's lantern. "No one can replace my father," she said, "but maybe one day someone will find it in their heart to care for me. A kind and honorable man. Someone like yourself, perhaps." A perfectly spherical tear trembled on her eyelash. There was nothing Ricky could do to stop his hand from wiping that tear away; it was as if all of humanity were pulling on a puppet string connected to his elbow and his wrist. As his sticky hand neared her face, her nostrils flared at the scent of the orange. Then her eyes widened as she saw the fleshy stands of fruit clinging to his fingers and thumb. She said, "Mister, was that my orange?" Ricky knew there was a great deal riding on his answer. It was like chaos theory: the wrong word here and the tremor might be felt all across Europe. Quick as a flash he produced the mangled orange from his pocket. "This?" he said. "Do you mean this? Oh, no, no, no. In England we call these apples. Apple. Try saying it after me. Apple. Apple."

RED DIRT
James Tate

An archeological team from a nearby university
asked my permission to dig in my backyard, and I said
no. They promised to restore my lawn to its current
state when finished, and I said no. They said the
university hadn't the money to offer me recompense, but
they personally were willing to offer me five thousand
dollars for my trouble, and I sad no. I didn't hear from
them after that. They never told me why my backyard held
such interest for them. And I didn't think to ask. I could
think about nothing else for months to come. Was there an
old Mayan city down there, or Incan, Etruscan, Viking?
It could be anything. I was sitting right on it. Some
nights it was almost too much to bear. I could hear the
screams of the sacrifices. I could see the jaguar god
stoically watching on his throne of gold. How was I supposed
to sleep? I couldn't tell anybody, and I couldn't call the
police. I didn't even want people coming to the house for
fear of the harm that might come to them. My friend thought
I had taken ill, and sent me baskets of fruit. And, I suppose,
I was sick in a way. I had lost my appetite, and I had grown
weak. The endless beheadings and mutilations had made me
numb. I had become a servant to the jaguar god, one of
thousands, of course, but I did get to come close enough
to him to see the serene beauty of his eyes. How could I
have ever doubted his cause. At night, I slept with the
other servants in an immense dormitory. We were as peaceful
as seraphim. When the winds blow, fine, red dirt sneaks in
and covers the floor. I dream we are being buried in it,

each day a little more. We go about our many duties, but
the dirt is inching up on us. In its way, it is beautiful,
the waves it makes, like the whistling of time. No one
mentions it. It's best this way. A peasant girl smiled
at me; then, she was gone.

HOTEL INSOMNIA
CHARLES SIMIC

I liked my little hole,
Its window facing a brick wall.
Next door there was a piano.
A few evenings a month
a crippled old man came to play
"My Blue Heaven."

Mostly, though, it was quiet.
Each room with its spider in heavy overcoat
Catching his fly with a web
Of cigarette smoke and revery.
So dark,
I could not see my face in the shaving mirror.

At 5 a.m. the sound of bare feet upstairs.
The "Gypsy" fortuneteller,
Whose storefront is on the corner,
Going to pee after a night of love.
Once, too, the sound of a child sobbing.
So near it was, I thought
For a moment, I was sobbing myself.

FROM "CHANG & ENG"

DARIN STRAUSS

This is an excerpt from the novel Chang & Eng, *the fictionalized story of the real-life Siamese twins for whom the term was coined. Chang and Eng—who were attached by a five-inch band at their chests—escaped Siam and came to America in the 1830s, where they achieved great fame, got caught up in the Civil War, married two sisters, and fathered twenty-one children.*

This scene shows us their wedding night, when the twins, who have never known physical affection of any kind, are to spend their first night with a woman. It having been agreed by coin flip that Chang and his bride Adelaide would have that first honeymoon night together in their three-person bedroom, Eng's wife Sarah goes to bed alone in a spare room, and Eng plans to attempt sleep.

As we decided to turn in, I said goodnight to my wife and leaned toward her, pulling Chang with me; I kissed her. I had given my lips to her before, at the wedding, with similar enthusiasm—tenderly, softly—but now it felt more familiar and I found myself importing visions of our future life together into the warmth of this first goodnight kiss. I divined the laughter of our unborn children, and the warmth of a thousand kisses to come, each to be more familiar that the last, and a crowd surged in my chest.

My bride pulled away, blinking. "Tomorrow," she said, wiping her lips on her forearm, turning to walk to her bedroom, swaying in a way that hit me physically. And then Chang, his wife Adelaide, and I went to the main bedroom and the riddles therein.

Adelaide went to freshen herself in the little wash basin next to the main bedroom, while Chang and I remained in the bedchamber and got into our usual rose pajamas, which we unbuttoned at our torsos to allow the band freedom and exposure. Chang wore his night-cap.

When Adelaide entered the room, lit only by the light of a single candle that she carried with her and the radiance of her nervous smile, Chang and I faced each other on our sides atop the bed—the only comfortable way for us to lie down. He fidgeted more than I. Adelaide placed the candle on the night table, and picked up a big hand mirror. She gazed into it while troubling with her hair, unable to disguise an aspect keenly curious and nearly panicked.

Chang's head trespassed on my pillow. His nose nearly touched mine. I felt the hurry of his heart. I tried to sleep, but it was difficult to keep my eyes closed now.

"I've often wondered what this moment would be like," my brother's wife was saying softly to her reflection. Eventually she placed the mirror face down on the dresser and shuffled toward us. "Maybe I'm wicked," she went on. "Ever since I was a girl I have been wondering . . . ."

My brother's wife glanced at me, then her eyes darted away amid the jerky disappearance and reappearance of her smile.

My brother's wife then let out a laugh she did not seem to trust. She tucked her blond hair behind her ears, but wisps fell about her cheeks and forehead. She crawled falteringly onto his side of the bed and, kneeling over her husband, she kissed his temple—not gently, or with any ease, but like a chicken bobbing after some feed.

Chang blinked his eyes. He said something, but his lips were too taut to shape the sound into a recognizable word.

"Maybe I'm wicked," she said. She reached for him.

I closed my eyes again—the method Chang and I had decided upon—to try becoming "mindless" for the next hour. If only I could fall asleep, I would not intrude on my twin's discretion. But with each bounce or jolt or kick of Adelaide's leg, my eyes opened instinctively, as if against my will.

Eyes closed tight again, hoping to find innocent thoughts, I could not ignore the substance that exists in men only to hasten the flow of blood at the sound of a woman giving herself for the first time. Her scent was light and poignant.

Yes, perhaps I could doze. I pictured the day's events and eased toward a dream. Adelaide's fingertips accidentally swiped my groin. Immediately, I found myself watching Chang lift her white frilled dressing gown, and, when my eyes were unfortunately opened again, he was taking off her white cotton undershorts and pulling her, naked, to him. We were on our backs, stretching the band. When Chang saw my eyes were opened, I shut them. Yes, I pictured the events of the day. Was that not how people brought on sleep? I seemed to have forgotten how one managed to fall off into slumber. After another trespass, a poke to my shinbone, I saw Adelaide sitting cross-legged over Chang, and unbuttoning the top of his pajamas and frowning. She had small breasts, very pale. The hair in the place where her lower body divided into her thighs looked like a dense furry valentine.

Now I really must sleep, I thought.

Her skin was lacking muscle, almost hairless; she was thin. I had not expected the naked female body to look like that, but it seemed perfect in its femininity, its weakness and oddity. After trying to close my eyes again, I felt a third unintentional brush of her hand—along my chest this time—as she fumbled with Chang's buttons, and again as she struggled to remove his red cloth pajamas. For a moment she stared directly at me, with soft eyes, just as scared as I was. Adelaide touched our connecting band hesitatingly, almost caressing it, a strange novelty.

She had pale breasts, I thought, very small.

I shut my eyes tight; I yawned, as if to encourage myself. Was I not tired? The sensation of her leg touching mine was faint and natural. Her throat was flecked with talcum powder.

Adelaide didn't look Chang in the face; she touched his chest, though, rubbed his skin, and she let loose a noise when she uncovered his manhood—she was shocked, likely, by the hair of Chang's pubis, which was (like mine) half black and half gray, divided vertically. And then my brother and his wife began to have relations.

Well, I asked myself, what had happened today? We had taken a carriage ride; I could think of that. The ride had been unpleasant and bouncy. Chang stirred me yet again; he was climbing on top of her and me. He was touching her breasts at the nipples, his mouth ajar, as if he feared he would never get the chance again. My arm was wrapped around Chang's shoulder, and to make this positioning possible, our band extended farther than it should go. The inopportune logistics meant that I had no choice but to curl against Adelaide, to cover her body partially—at the curve of her hip—and move along her leg as my brother rocked back and forth. I really should try leaving them alone, I thought. Chang caught me looking; he turned away quickly, as did I.

After some rolling of the three of us, Adelaide's soft blond hair came tickling across my neck, simultaneously gift and ordeal. I strained to keep my eyes shut as knees, elbows, fingers poked and bounced off of me. Our band ached. Though my eyes were closed, I knew she was still on top of my brother because her hair gladdened my neck once again. I let my stare glide over her coloring face, following the swerve of bone in her exquisite cheek. Another accident, her fingers ran involuntarily against my palms before she could withdraw her embarrassed hand. She was alarmed and self-conscious and nearly crying. I felt alone and exposed.

Meanwhile Chang, his eyes closed, perspired, bit his lip, and then began triumphantly to smile; suddenly I felt something, too, like a feather lightly dragged across the length of my body, chin to feet, and I shivered. I began gradually, instinctually, I hoped imperceptibly, to approach the cheeks of my brother's bride with my own lips opened in an O. I cut their journey short at the last moment. The wind made a shrill noise through the magnolias outside, and the mattress sounded its own creaky song.

That was it. Yes, I eyed my brother's bride now, sleep be damned, and I hoped to see in her a new knowledge. I assumed that by seeing her naked I would be able somehow to comprehend everything about this woman—to locate the secret that made her an individual, and to draw out what was essential about her. But of course I could not contain anything at all about this woman, just the opposite. It might as well have been ten Adelaides I saw now. The one sister-in-law as ten-headed mystery.

When she and my brother were finished, it took Chang a moment to separate himself from his wife. He was panting like a mackerel plucked into the air. And then Adelaide, smiling, was covering Chang's mouth with her tiny hand, resting her head on his breast, and staring back at me.

I assumed I would be unable to fall asleep for some time.

INSOMNIA

Frank Stack

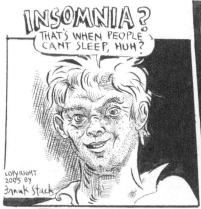

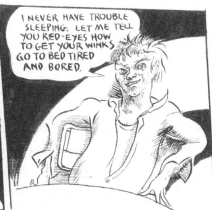

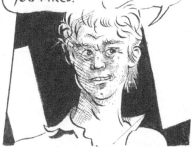

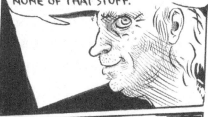

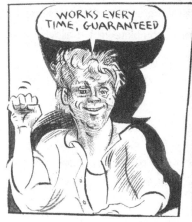

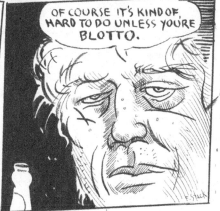

SELECTIONS FROM "LETTERS TO WENDY'S"
Joe Wenderoth

TELL US ABOUT YOUR VISIT ...

December 17, 1996
The factory pulls its sleepy lovers into a dirty "area." Sleep-aids are manufactured. Sleep almost comes to those who can afford it. The pornographer decides what to do. The "actors" say they understand. Big lights are hauled in and arranged around a couch. The couch is not special. The "actors" are not acting. The factory feels betrayed, steps up production. The "actors" can almost sleep now.

February 26, 1997
so troubling is the lull in this carriage that the authorities have outnumbered themselves and required that the seasons repeat their intentions until they are less meaningless than the colors for which they rush—so spectacular is the comfort of the seat that the authorities are able to overlook the seasons' failure to meet requirements and to feel the meaningless rush as an impromptu massage.

May 19, 1997
The thriving banks of fluorescence. No withdrawals here—only the useless growth of interest. I feel good about the establishment of complete light. It allows me to course fully dangling into the given accident. So much argument over what's truly *given*, the dangling or the accident that severs it. What really matters is the coursing, which is not given, but taken.

June 8, 1997
The present hidden by a hurting heap—only laceration pleases it, prepares it for ne-glect—I'm the nothing-blade in the hurting heap—I drag sleep by the hair until it

speaks—I don't hear what it says—I'm the hurting heap with the nothing-blade sleeping me apart—I am prepared for neglect—I am prepared for nothing but neglect

June 12, 1997

HELP! (this helmet is fusing with my skull)

June 19, 1997

Pain and sleep and dull flocks of noise stitching them together with what flesh there is. Notice how deep the flocks carry the needle into one and then the other. One gets the impression it will fall all apart in time. And though quite impossible to believe, this impression is nevertheless the whole truth.

June 23, 1997

Mumb-drool erections smothering Attention at the behest of a towering devouring one-time-only Sleeping Face. Smothering predictably—they are indeed drool—but at the same time with a quickness, an ability to found themselves, already erect, in the fictive interior, causing the invaluable embarrassment of its sudden debut. (There is a fry on the floor)

July 16, 1997

The surgery lasting much longer than expected. I guess we sleep standing up, we surgeons. We sing softly to ourselves, if not to the patient. What use singing to the patient? We sing about not being able to tell day from night. We sing about closing up the body and going home. We sing in our sleep. The surgery seems further from an end, now, than it ever has before.

July 26, 1997

Now I lay me down to teeth—I drain the gruel my hole to keep—and if I should die before I quake—I say the drain my hole to take. Now I lay me down to feet—I brain the air my pain to treat—and if I should fuck before I wake—I sprain the eye my soul to take. (I pray bring me a softer booth!)

THURSDAY

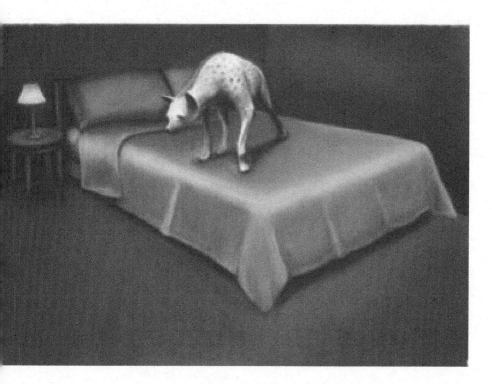

Possibly an Animal

FRIENDS WHO WEREN'T THERE
MATTHEW ROHER

Unseasonably warm, & sick, no sleep.
My teeth held themselves all night like a beast's
with my mouth closed, I could see them. They weren't
broken or dreaming. I lay there talking
amiably with my friends who weren't there.
The whole house shuddered & bitter sickness
smells like bitter tea. My wife fitfully
clawing me in sleep, a fire in my ears.
That word you always say, I don't know what
it means but it sounds pretty. Medicine
crashes upon the shore. I wonder if
I will be reassuring company
to myself when I die? I must get out
of bed right away and work towards that end.

A STATE OF VARIANCE
AIMEE BENDER

On her fortieth birthday, the woman lost the ability to sleep for more than a single hour. She did not accumulate a tired feeling; in fact, that one hour served the purpose of eight, and she awoke refreshed. But because that hour was full of only the most intense, involving sleep, the sleep beyond rapid eye movement, the only consequence was that she had no time in her sleep hours for dreams. And so, during the day, she would experience moments when the rules of the world would shift and she would see, inside her tea kettle, a frog floating, dead. And then blink and it would be gone. Or she would greet the mailman and he would hand her a basket of sea water, dripping, with stamps floating wetly on top. And then she would smile and bring in the mail. These moments sprinkled throughout every day; she still had a driver's license and wondered if she should revoke it herself, as the zombies who passed through the crosswalk and disappeared into the lamppost were confusing.

She assumed she would die at eighty. She figured this because the sleep shift began on her fortieth birthday and all her life, things had happened symmetrically like that. Her birthdate was 11.25.52 and that was not notable until she realized that she had been born in Amsterdam and there the day comes first: 25.11.52; the address of the only house she could afford for miles and miles was 1441, on a street named Circle Road on the edges of Berkeley. She had a son the day her father died. Her son's face was almost a perfect mirror of itself, in such a way that one realized how imperfections created trust because no one trusted her son, with that perfect symmetry in his face; contrary to the articles that stated that women would orgasm easily above him, beneath him, due to that symmetry, no—his symmetry was too much, and women shied away, certain he was a player. Certain he would dump them. And because no one approached him, when he did have a girlfriend every now and again he *would* dump them, because he found he did not trust them either, because they were always looking at him so furtively—making, with their faces, the action of holding up your hands in front of your chest to block a blow. He told his mother he could not seem to meet a woman that had a core strength to her, and his mother, studying geometry at the kitchen table with cut-outs of triangles and squares, said she was sorry for what her pregnancy had done.

"What did it do?" he asked.

She held a mirror up to his nose. He saw his face in the hinged reflection. "What?" he said. Then she did it to herself, and the sight of his mother in perfect symmetry so disturbed him that he made himself a huge ham sandwich.

"So what are you saying?" he asked, mouth full of food.

"I am saying that your face repels trust," she said. "Because it is too exact. I am saying," she told him, "that I will die on my eightieth birthday, because I stopped sleeping at forty."

He knew, in a vague way, about the sleeping. The shapes on the table danced in front of her and slipped into her mouth, large mints. Then they were regular again. The mirror on the table was a mouth. She put a finger in it and it bit her, wet. She'd finally told her son about the sleeping when he complained that she had made him too many colorful crocheted blankets and he had no more room for them in his apartment. "Take them to the shelter," he'd pleaded, and then asked, "how are you making all these anyway? Are you taking drugs?" (He himself had been taking drugs to take the edge off how he felt when he smiled at another person who seemed to have an inordinately tough time smiling back.) His mother had laughed. She told him not about the dreaming aspect but about the one hour, the way she didn't feel tired, and how it began promptly on her fortieth birthday.

He finished his sandwich and touched the blob of mustard left on the plate with the bed of his fingertip.

"Are you saying you believe in some kind of grand plan?" he asked. "Because I never thought you raised me to believe in that kind of overarching concept."

He returned to the refrigerator and popped open a ginger ale.

"I'm just noticing the patterns," she said. "If I live past my eightieth birthday, well then."

"Well then," he said. "I sure hope you do."

"Mmm." But her voice was so doubtful that he made a mental note to be sure to be there on that day itself, so that she would not try to do anything herself, so interested in the pattern that she might let herself be a sacrifice to it.

Neither missed their father/husband who traveled so often he was unrecognizable when he returned. He came back from the latest trip with his hair dyed black and a deadly cough that landed him in the hospital. He lay there for weeks and weeks, and his hair grew in long and brown. The cough got worse. Above him, before death, stood his symmetrical son, whom even he did not trust, and his wife who he could not sleep next to anymore, as she read until all hours and wanted to talk to him and had forgotten that other people needed more than an hour. She resented the world, he felt, resented that all people were not exactly like her in this way. She was so lonely for those seven hours, and when he awoke he always felt that she was slightly blaming him for sleeping. After she turned forty, he traveled more, so that those eight hours could be his alone, and in different cities he loved different beds—his mistresses not flesh and blood but made of pillows and sheets and the wide open feeling of waking up without alarm or expectation. As he died, as he looked at these two people he loved most, he only thought: what a curious pair they are, aren't they? and then was the white light, and he felt fine about succumbing to it. He was not, by nature, a big fighter.

A year or so after his father died, the son felt a strong desire to get his mother a suitor, so that his mother would not lean on him too much as the main man in her life. He knew a son's role could be confused that way, just as he'd felt the tugging from inside all those crocheted blankets, and he was too keenly vulnerable himself to the attention. He could see it, marriage to Mom, never official or blessed, and yet as implicit as breakfast or dinner. He did not want that. For all the lack of trust the world had bestowed upon him, he still had hope that somehow he'd get a scar or a sore eye or something would happen to his face that would soften its appearance to others, and allow him into the palm of true love. So he went on a dating search for his mother. He answered several personal ads for men who were looking for women that sounded, more or less, like her, and so he wrote them, explaining that he was looking for his mother, and invited them, one by one, over to the house on Circle Road, under the guise of tutor. The men were skeptical about the idea, which seemed untrustworthy, and even more skeptical once they met the kid, who seemed untrustworthy, but they all fell for his mother, almost elegantly, and in con-trast to the general lore that good men were difficult to find, here were four, almost instantly, who were ready to take her mourning and knead it into their hearts. Two became her weekend companions: one on Sunday day, one on Friday evening. She did not tell them of the sleeping, or of how when watching a movie, how another movie often superimposed itself onto the screen so that when he asked, after, how she'd liked it, she wasn't sure which movie he had seen and which was her dream addition.

The son, now, had some space to do things. His father was gone. Which was sad but his father had never trusted him, and that had always been a problem. He went to the coffee shop down the street from his apartment in Oakland and ordered himself a raisin scone and a black tea. Then he sat down at the table of a large man, a man with tattoos but the old kind, before tattoos became dainty and about spiritual life. This man wore tattoos from the time when tattoos meant you liked to kick people around.

"Yes?" the man said, moving his newspaper aside.

The son didn't move. He sipped his coffee.

"I'm sitting here?" said the man. He was a big man too. He took up most of the table. There were plenty of other free tables in the cafe. The young man trembled inside but he kept his hand steady. He steadied his symmetrical face.

"You a homo or something?" asked the man.

The son didn't respond. But he could see the man digesting the face, the perfect face, and the man lifted the table gently, and the scone slid down into the boy's lap, and the tea wobbled, and the boy just put the scone back on the now slanted table and kept his eyes on the scrawny facial hair of the man.

The man, Marty, was tired. He did not want to fight. He had done that so many times before. He was tired of it, and he was taking classes now, and they told him to acknowledge how he was really hurt inside, not angry at all. He read his paper high over his head and stopped looking at the young man. So, it was a homo. So, he was picked up today at the cafe by a homo. This was new for him. He decided to do what that lady said, and try to find the humor in it, and when he did he really did find it funny and behind his paper, he started to laugh.

Well, the young man was stuck. He'd wanted a hit, a real hit, a hit that would complicate his face. Finally he put a hand on the man's newspaper, folding it down. "Listen," he said. "I'm sorry to bother you, but I just want to get hit." Marty laughed and laughed some more. His arm tattoo read Skull Keeper, and had an illustration of bones wrapped in ribbons. "You want to get hit?" he said. "Too bad. I'm done with that shit."

"Please?" said the young man, and Marty said no, but the tight businessman eavesdropping at the next table with an iced mocha blend said he'd do it, sure, a hit?

"Right on the cheek," said the young man, and he asked Marty to oversee because now he trusted Marty far more than the tight businessman whose smile was too pleased at the idea. "Let's all go out back? Please?" he asked Marty, who folded up his paper and agreed, because it was the modern world, and he was old but open-minded and being the protector was a better role for him anyway, maybe a role to consider, in fact, for the future. And the tight businessman looked so tightly delighted and the boy said, "cheek please," but he did not know the tight business-man had poor centering perception, and had never, in fact, hit another man although he'd wanted to, his whole life, ever since he had been teased everyday on the walk to school by that bastard boy, Adam Vermouth, who had told him in a squawking voice that he was useless, useless, useless. The tight businessman played with his hands as fists all the time at the office, but when put in the actual situation, aiming for the cheek, what he got instead was the nose, and he slammed the boy straight on and broke the bone, blood pouring out of his nostrils. "Okay?" said Marty, hold-ing his arms out flat like a referee. "Are we done?" "That's good," gasped the boy, reeling with pain, and the tight businessman was just warming up, was dancing on his toes, ready to pummel this handsome young man into the brick of the cafe's back wall, but Marty clamped one soft big paw on the businessman's shoulder, and said, "You're done now, son." The tight businessman relaxed under Marty's hand, and the young man, too, relaxed under Marty's voice, and later, Marty did decide that it had been a far better day for him, being the fight mediator, the protective bulldog, and when he told the lady he had figured something out, tears broke into his eyes, like eggs cracking, bright and fresh. She was proud of him. He was such a good man inside, underneath all the butt kicking and bravado.

The young man, bleeding all over the wall, waved off offers to go to the hospital or the doctor. "No, thank you, thank you," he said, stumbling inside, using up a pile of brown recycled napkins, then holding the cafe's one pint of coffee ice cream to his nose, and the businessman kept saying, "it will heal poorly," and the young man said that was the point. And he shook the hand of the tight businessman who was feeling cheated that the fight was so short, like a taste of nectar one could hardly even feel in the mouth. The young man waved at Marty, who was at the payphone telling about his revelation, and he headed home. There, he tended to his nose for days, hoping and hoping, and he went over to his mother's on the day he was ready to really look at it straight on, ready to remove the band-aids making a little pattern all over his face. She was in the kitchen, eating jelly beans off the counter, and she helped him peel each one off, one at a time, and then they both went to the bath-room mirror. They stared at his face for a long, long time.

What had happened is that it healed symmetrically. The nose was severely broken and bumpy, but the bump was a symmetrical band over the middle of his nose.
It had complicated the vertical planes of his face, but horizontally, he still matched
himself exactly. The young man's eyes filled and he felt the despair rushing into his
throat, but his mother, wiping his cheeks clear of the leftover crusted blood, listened
to the story and laughed, and said, "Son, my sweet, sweet son, it's just that you are
a butterfly. That's just what you are. I don't think you can do anything about it."

Finally, he was eating a hamburger one afternoon and when licking the ketch-
up off the knife, he cut open the side of his lip. It was a small mark, but it needed
stitches, and when they took out the stitches he had a small raised area above
the left side of his lip which provided the desperately needed window. He met a
woman—Sherrie Marla—in a week. True, about a month later, she, while kissing
him passionately, bit the other side, creating an identical mark. She dabbed ice on
his lip, apologizing, and he dreaded it, dreaded her change, his eyes filling with tears
in advance of her leaving, but the fact was Sherrie Marla trusted him already. When
he took the ice off, and showed to her his new symmetry, she didn't flinch. His face
was him to her now; it was not a map or an indicator of some abstract idea. Turned
out it was only the first impression he'd needed to alter.

In bed, she turned to him with bright eyes, touching his lip wound with her
fingertips, her head propped on her open hand.

"You have movie star lips now," Sherrie Marla told him, smiling, as he leaned in
to kiss her, tenderly, her own kisses very very gentle on the sore area, just pillows
in the air between them.

Her own face was wildly asymmetrical. One eye much higher than the other.
A nostril tilted. The smile lopsided. The front right tooth chipped. The dented chin.
The larger right breast. The slightly gnarled foot. It had caused her her own share
of problems. We are all, generally, symmetrical: ants, elephants, lions, fish, flowers,
leaves. But she was a tree. No one expects a tree to be symmetrical at all. It opens
its arms, in its unevenness, and he, the butterfly, flew inside.

ON GETTING THE SHEETS TO STAY ON THE BED . . .

JOSHUA COHEN

. . . it's impossible, mad, the sheets are always coming off the bed, rather the bed is always coming off up from under the sheets, off: up: under: anyway, one never stays on or off the other, the two rarely, if never, commingle in perfection: you, me, you're always kneeling on one edge, stretching the sheet, fitted, over another edge opposite or diagonal it can't, won't, reach because you're kneeling on that very edge that would give it enough slack, enough sheet, fitted, to fit, perfectly, the sheet, flat, mussed too, in a pile at your feet or else off the bed entirely, massed forgotten on the floor, you're always readjusting and adjusting, pulling one side to push the other, push-pulling, making taut to obtain slack, slackening to taut an other edge, the bunch, the corner, half on, off half, it's a mess, a burden, unnecessary, especially when you know, you're sure, that in your sleep you'll—unconsciously, subconsciously—toss-turn the sheets awry again, away and off, yet again and again again as always, dreaming all the while that the bed it's less a bed than it is an ocean, the ocean (your sheets are blue, mine are), and that the sheets themselves they're the ocean's water, waters, the surface and the surface under underneath the surface, the depth, depths rising and writhing, falling into wake, and that no amount/degree/work/hope will ever help, or succeed, in mating the two waters above and below that God created before He slept, too.

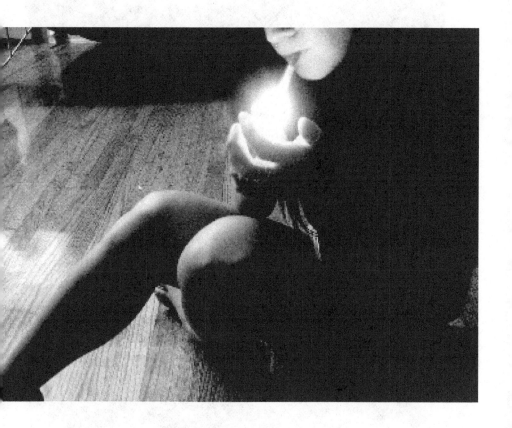

ANOTHER SLEEPLESS NIGHT
CRICKET SUICIDE

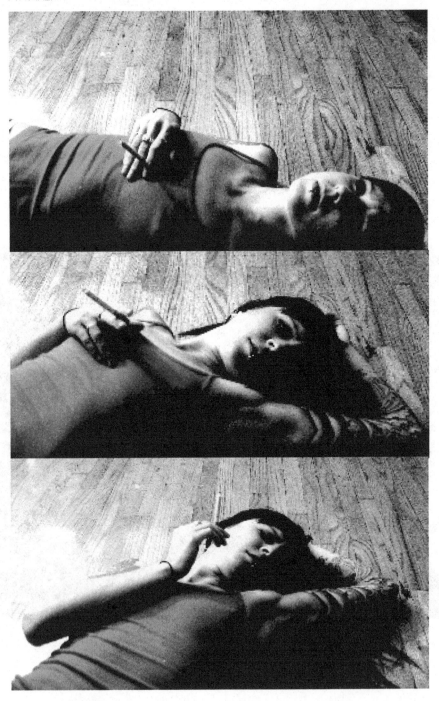

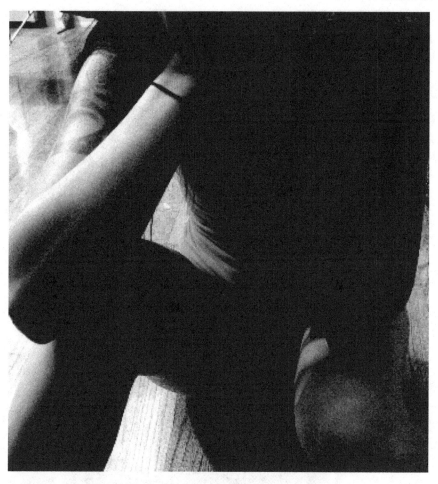

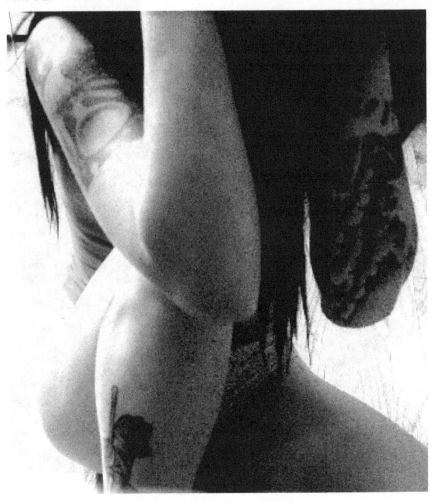

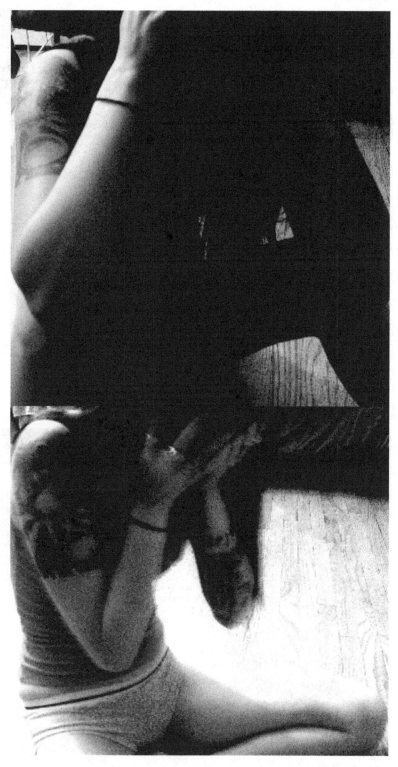

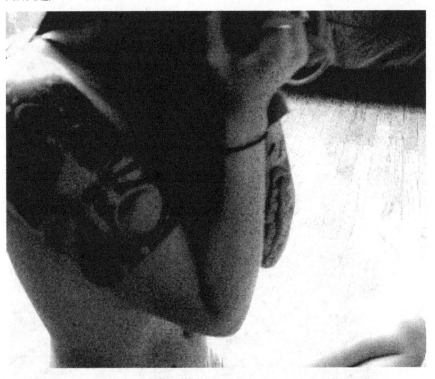

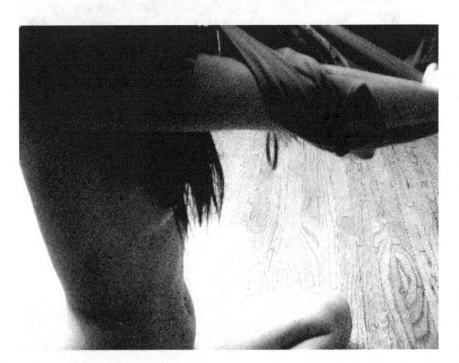

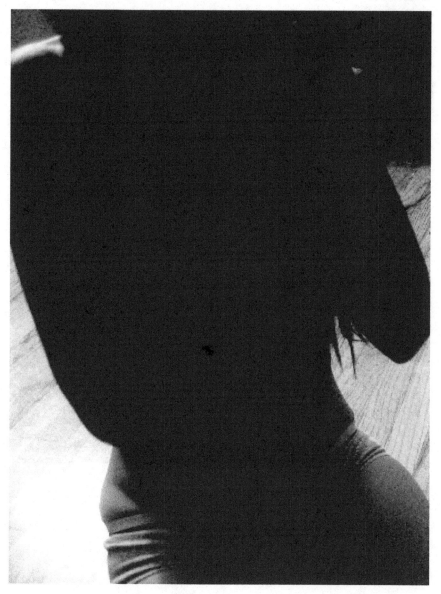

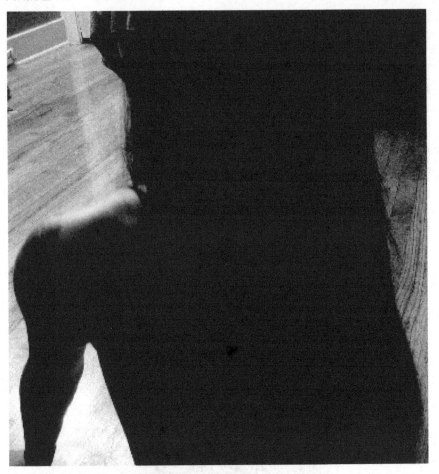

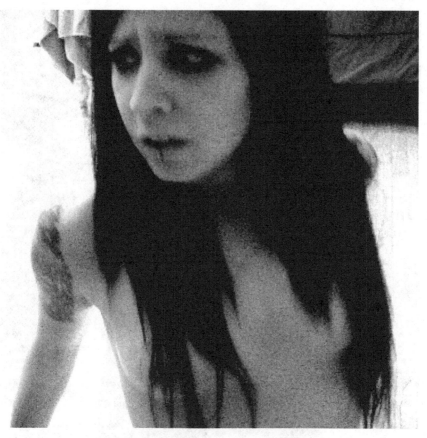

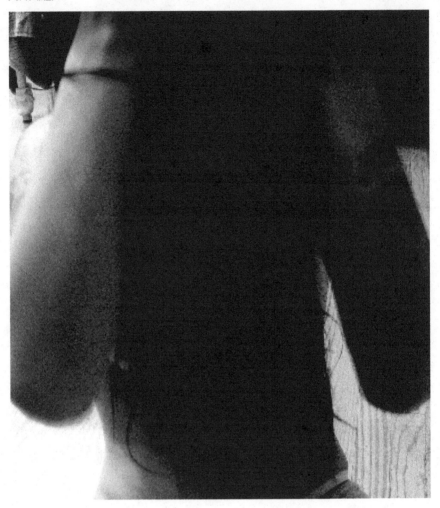

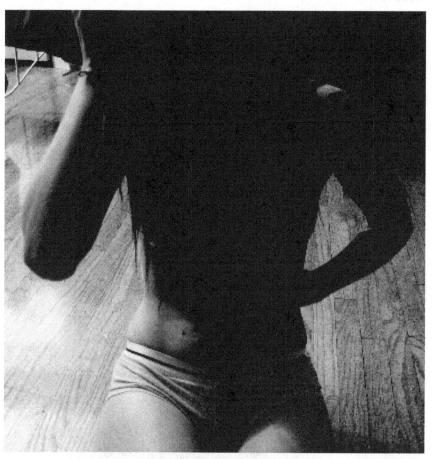

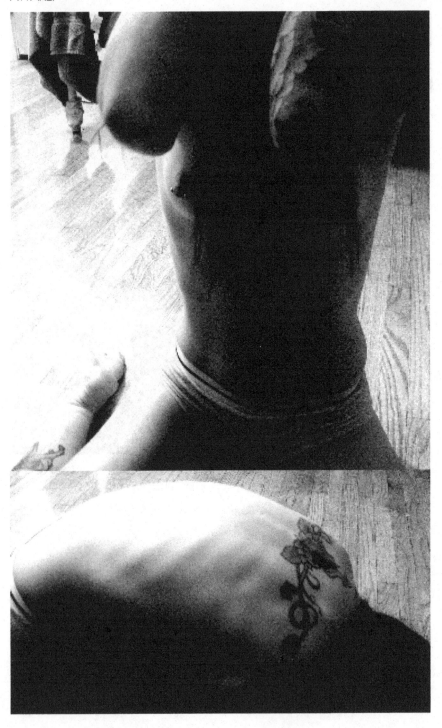

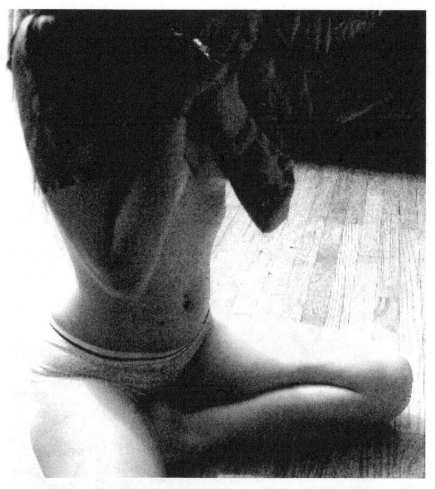

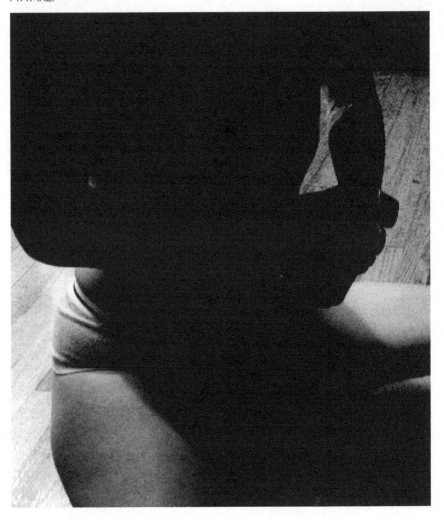

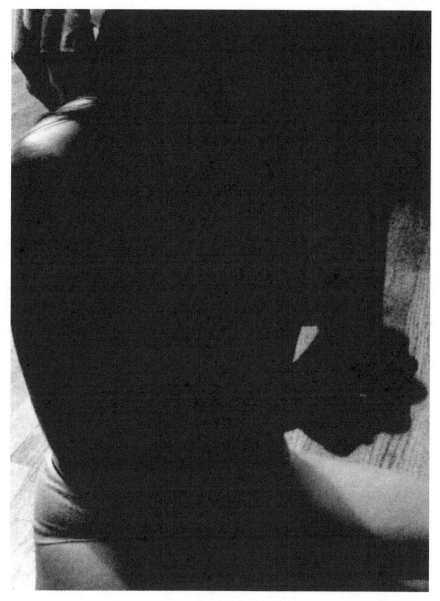

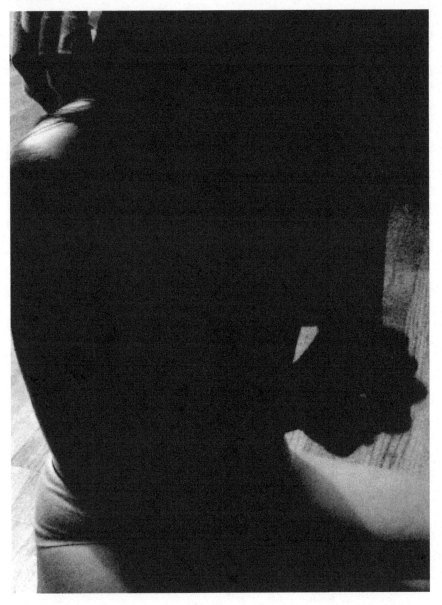

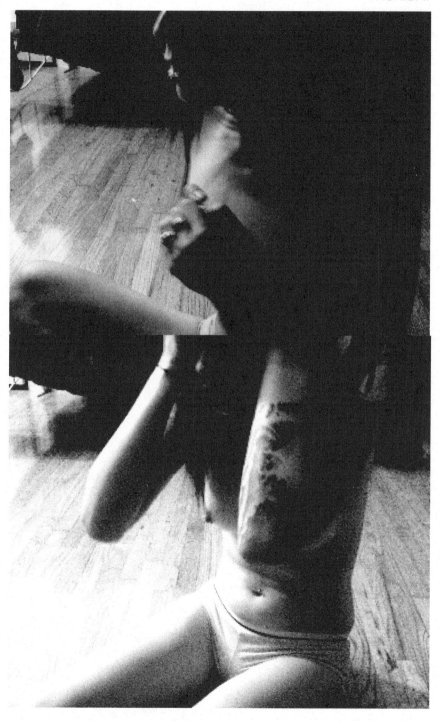

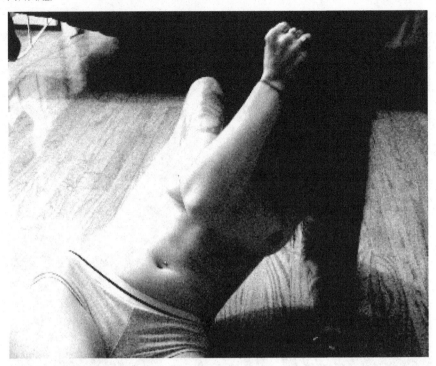

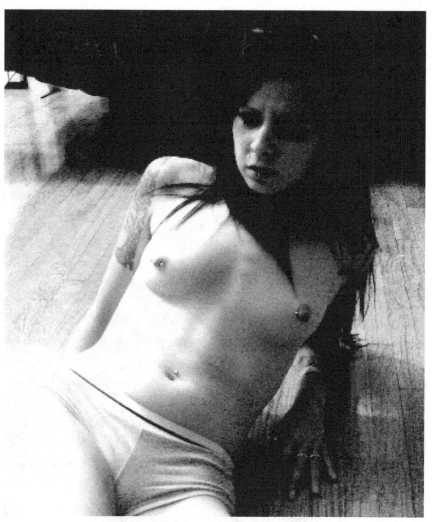

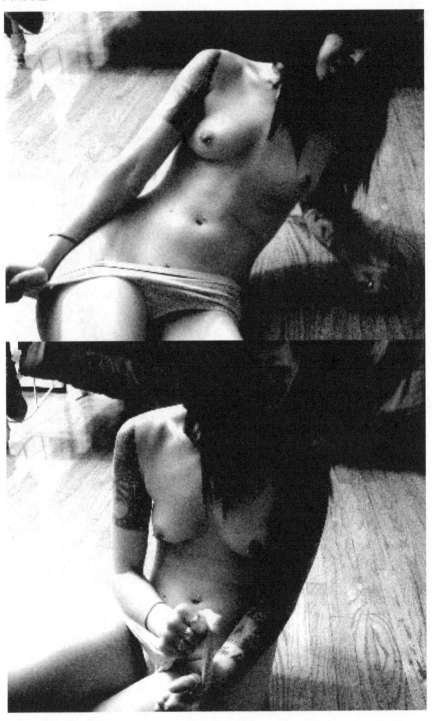

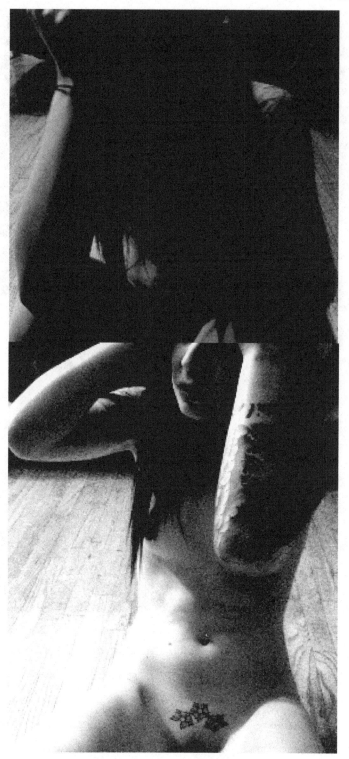

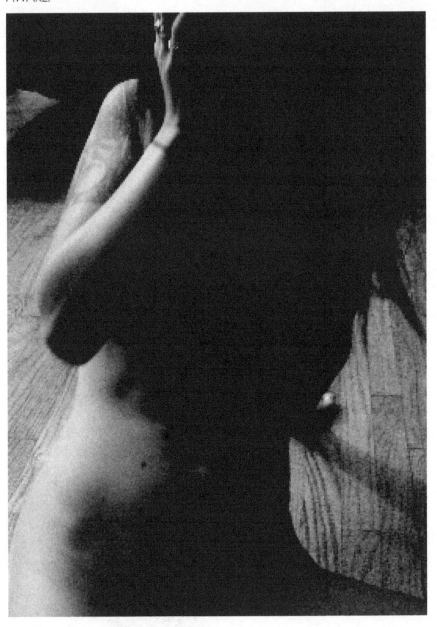

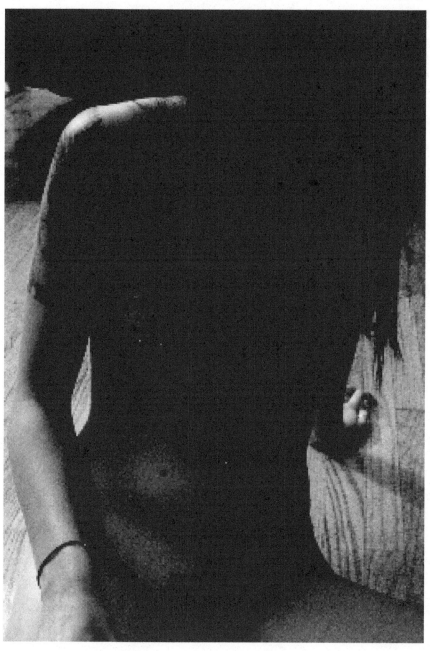

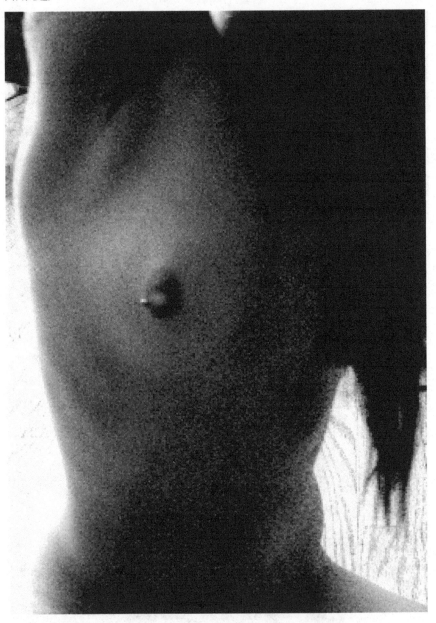

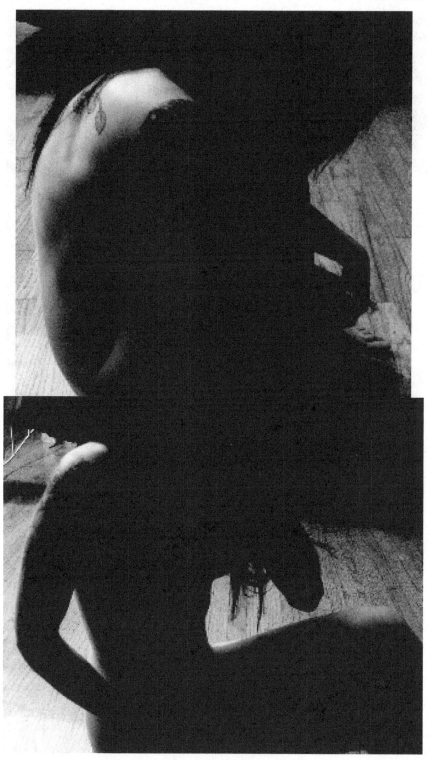

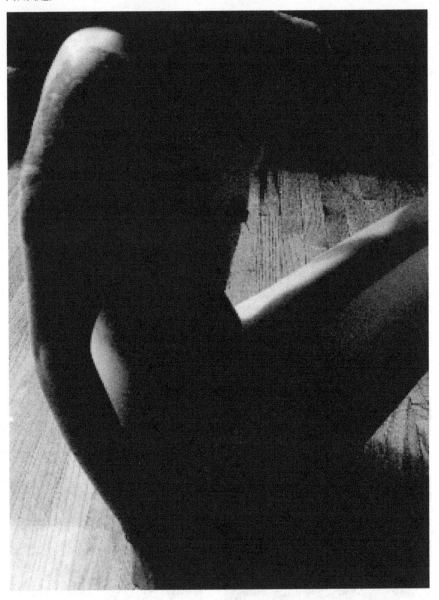

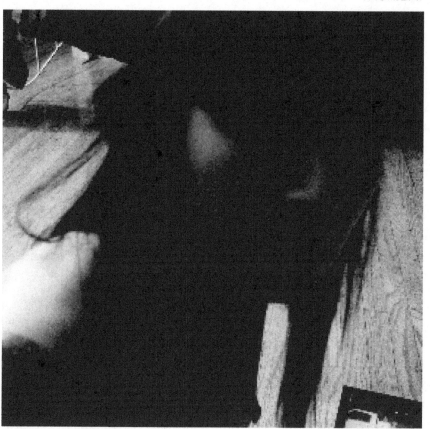

IN THE INSOMNIAC NIGHT
Joyce Carol Oates

In the night in the insomniac night she lies in her bed whispering *Sleep, sleep!* But she isn't listening listening instead to the sweet-mournful beat of the frothy briny greeny-bitter waves at the ocean's edge a half-mile away in the night in the wind-buffeted liquidy moonlight spilling through partly closed venetian blinds onto the faded-wallpaper wall and a wedge of plaster ceiling shaped like an isosceles triangle floating. Moonlight calling to her, teasing. A man's face winking out of the moon. *Where are your children?* the voice asks pleasantly and her reply is immediate and easy *Both are here beneath this roof, asleep in their beds safe in the night miles from all harm.* For children are not inhabitants of the insomniac night. Children know nothing of the insomniac night. Sleeping deeply and innocently in ignorance. Holly who is eight, Mark who is five. Fatherless children. Yet happy children. Happy children because fatherless. *Both beneath this roof in their rooms close by my own and tomorrow Sunday: church.* In the old life of the city amid traffic, poison-exhaust, sirens renting the air like razor wire, there had been no church, not a thought of *church, faith, God, community, Jesus meek and Jesus mild.* And she herself non-believing, a skeptic. Yes and embarrassed. In the city in the old life. In the old life in the marriage. But the old life is past, is fled. Escaped. The old life is gone. Now the new life in the seaside town in the neat attractive stone-and-stucco slightly shabby bungalow on a street of similar bungalows inland from the ocean. Rented, leased in her name. In her name exclusively. Legally. Now the divorce is final, the custody suit settled. Mostly in her favor though of course the father, the ex-husband, has certain visitation rights. But now the children are in her care beneath a roof provided for them by her, by the mother. By this woman who astonished with her unexpectedly fierce, possessive love for her children like a lioness's for her cubs. She who had not seemed to herself as to others an inordinately maternal woman. But now this new life this new adventure *Once upon a time, a very special time, there was a mommy and a little girl and a little boy who came to live in a town near the Atlantic Ocean where it was said nothing had happened in a hundred years that was not something happy, a happy sur-*

prise. Except these nights, these autumn nights awake hearing the wind in the pines and the ragged clouds blown overhead scratching the pearly sky, hearing the *beat beat beat* of the waves against the pebbly shore that stir an old ache in her loins, an old weakness she would have wished to believe she'd overcome. Softly begging *Sleep! Oh please* for consciousness exhausts her, her weeks are strenuous bouts of commuting seventy miles to work, seventy miles back home, on weekends sleep is precious to her *Try to sleep! for God's sake! what is wrong with you, Judith!* even as her heart beats with a sullen stubbornness and her feet kick the bedclothes *I don't want to sleep, God damn I want to run to fly through the night. Where the night will take me.* Her long slenderly muscled runner's legs like the legs of a young horse primed to run, to run, to run. But she can't give in! Lying arms crossed still as the figure on the prow of a ship. Lying still willing herself *Sleep!* for she is a single mother now, she must behave like an adult woman of thirty-two and not the irresponsible restless girl the girl she is. Insomnia is a weakness to be overcome as she has overcome other weaknesses. Insomnia is not in her nature. In the old life in the city in the failing miserable marriage to a man now a stranger to her were shameful sedative nights, sweaty oblivion nights of no dreams and by morning a mouth parched as if blistered and dazed headachy hours when for no reason her eyes leaked tears so Holly bit at her thumbnail *Mommy why are you crying?* and Mark pushed against her with his scared puny whine *Mommy! stop that!* But drugged sleep was not in her nature either. Nothing of weakness in her character is in fact her character. Except *I want to be out outside, to run, to fly through the night where the night will take me.*

Finally then she gives in. Kicks off the bedcovers, rises and dresses swiftly, fastens her hair into a ponytail, puts on her running shoes. Her breath quickening like a child's on the verge of an adventure. *Only for a half-hour* checking her watch which she wars night and day, rarely removes *back by 1:40 a.m.* This is the second time this week unless it's the third time she will slip away from the house too restless to too alert and yearning to sleep. How many times since moving to this quiet seaside town out of the old exhausting life of the city several months before. She ties the slightly frayed laces of the running shoes with mounting excitement, an anticipation of pleasure. Shoes that fit her long narrow feet so perfectly: like a caress. She smiles to think how ironic how funny: these waterstained not-new shoes feel to her more loving than any man cupping her feet in his hands had ever been.

*

She'd several times glimpsed him following her with his eyes. Tracking her with his eyes. In town, once at the mini-mart. This place new to her at the edge of the ocean: Edgewater, New Jersey. A local handyman probably. Manual laborer judging by his walnut-dark skin. Carved-looking face. Black hair that looked smudged as tar. He was of less than average height for an adult man but compactly, solidly built. Thick neck. Upper body development like a boxer. Legs rather short, though by no means stunted. A muggy September day he'd been wearing a t-shirt that fitted his chest tightly and khaki shorts, unusually short shorts for a man. Hard sinewy muscled thighs. Legs and arms covered in dark hairs that appeared imbricated, like an animal's pelt. His eyes easing upon her as she kept in motion, not slowing to look around. *Never make eye contact with a stranger especially a strange man* she'd gently cautioned both her children. Oh she couldn't be certain the walnut-dark man had actually been watching her, each of the several times was the sort of situation where you can't be certain. So simply ignore. Forget. In the corner of an eye. Watching? Can't know so wisest not to imagine. Not to alarm. She was not an excitable woman, not any longer. Here in Edgewater, New Jersey, population 1,470. The seaside town with the pebbly beaches unlike most of the Jersey shore, not very popular with summer tourists. A place where nothing has happened in a long time, the real estate woman remarked shaking her head. Median age fifty-nine and rising. Great place to bring up children, of course. The last time she'd seen the walnut-dark man, the man with the carved face and swath of tar for hair, she'd been hurrying to her car parked at the curb in front of the post office. Holly and Mark were in the car, a Saturday morning of errands in this new town at the edge of the Atlantic Ocean where there was always a wind, always the briny smell of the estuary. And each errand pleasurable in itself. *This is our life now, our life the three of us in Edgewater, New Jersey.* Where the children's father when he came every third weekend to take them away, Friday morning to Sunday evening, was an outsider, a temporary visitor not at ease as in the city in the old life. After the post office was the dry cleaner's then the video shop another time to rent "Pocahontas" then Oleander Farm at the outskirts of town where there was apple slush, cinnamon doughnuts, a mule and goats and a Shetland pony and many cats for the children to pet. So she hadn't given a second thought to the walnut-dark man on the sidewalk tracking her with his eyes.

Nor thinking at that time, of course, that there might be any connection between him and the lead-colored Chrysler van. That looked as if it might have been a workingman's van once, sides now crudely painted over. There was a crescent moon in silver on the driver's door, not very skillfully rendered. She'd seen this vehicle once or twice in town without taking any special notice of it except casually *Why is it parked there, motor running? for so many minutes?* while she'd been in the drug store patiently waiting for the elderly pharmacist to fill a prescription. In the whitish glare of hot autumn the lead-colored van's windshield. was blinding, she couldn't see who sat behind the wheel or whether in fact there was anyone behind the wheel, at all.

*

Quietly she checks the children in their bedrooms. The bungalow is a single sto-ry with an unfinished attic, her bedroom and theirs at the rear of the house. Next to her bedroom is Mark's, not much larger than a walk-in closet. But a cozy com-fortable room whose walls she'd painted herself, cornflower blue. And the luminous Mother Goose plastic night light on the floor, reassuring should the child wake with a start not knowing where he is. In the townhouse in the city *We don't want to coddle Mark, spoil him* the children's father had warned. *He will only see that darkness holds no terrors if he can experience darkness for himself.* But she is the mother, it is she who makes decisions now. So the luminous Mother Goose burns nightly in a corner of the five-year-old's room. Where is the harm? no harm certainly. And how hard Mark is sleeping! as he'd done as an infant in the crib: Sunk in sleep so he seems scarcely to be breathing and his skin clammy-pale as if his body's heat has been sucked inside by the tension of his pumping heart and organs. In that region of dreams to which his mother leaning above his bed has no entrance, knows herself excluded. *Love I love you Mark-y, baby Mark-y.* She dares to bend closer brushing her lips against his warm forehead and dares to tug up the blanket beneath his chin. Mark doesn't wake of course, he sleeps so soundly. Next is Holly in her bed in her room across the hall from Mommy's bedroom, asleep too, silky pale-gold hair like her mother's at that age but resembling her father in the set of the eyes, set of the chin. Her daughter her miraculous first-born. Out of what starry dust, what maze of unnamable un-countable atoms. Out of what unknowable void. *What do babies dream?* the mother had asked as Holly, as an infant, fell asleep nursing, and twitched and flailed her tiny fattish arms clearly enthralled by some sort of dream. And Holly's father had said *Obviously, babies don't dream, can't dream lacking memory and language. No more than an animal can dream.* And the mother who was a new, young mother bold and giddy and flirtatious and in love at that time with the baby and with the baby's father and with herself such a success had laughed *How do you know, do you remember?* and he'd said with a smile but in finality *No of course I don't remember, haven't I said babies have no memory. Our daughter's brain is an emptiness ready to be filled.*

Holly is now eight years old, a third grader. Beautiful child if at times touch-me-not. High-strung. Quick to tears, quick to rages. But she loves her mother, hugs her mother tight a dozen times a day. *Mommy I love you Mommy when can I have a kitten?* At Oleander Farm there are kittens to be adopted, but not just now. Holly's room is a little-girl's room the two of them had decorated together, sunflower curtains, pumpkin-colored shag rug, white plastic glow-in-the dark Kitty Clock on the bureau. Her mother doesn't dare lean over to kiss Holly, Holly is a notoriously light sleeper. A frown flickering over her face in profile on the pillow like ripples on the surface of water. Again thinking as she backs out of the room, shuts the door silently *What do children dream?* feeling a stab of jealousy for never will she know.

*

Of course the windows to the children's rooms are locked, and the blinds drawn neatly to the window sills. Every night without fail. Double locks on both the front and rear doors of the house though there is virtually no crime here in Edgewater, New Jersey.

Where's the harm? No one will know. In sweater, slacks, running shoes slipping outside through the kitchen door and locking it, the key wrapped in a tissue in her pocket for safekeeping. She will not run far, or long. In the night in the wind-buffeted insomniac night her route has been a rectangle of which the approximate center is the stone-and-stucco bungalow on Spruce Street, the children sleeping in their beds.

Her heart quickens in rapture: running!

What freedom, what bliss: running!

Out through the carport, out the narrow asphalt driveway and to the street and along the street of darkened houses in softened leaves lining the gutters and the fresh fragrance of the leaves stirred by her running feet, her heart beginning to beat strong and hard as a fist, confident in its rhythm, this speed matches her metabolism, this is the true rhythm of her being, this is where she belongs not lying in bed beneath smothering covers trying to sleep not helpless not a passive cringing frightened woman: no longer. Running in the night in chill autumnal moonlight smelling of the estuary, of the ocean. *This is my life, no one can deny me my life, I am not a mother only, I am a woman before I am a mother and I was a girl before I was a woman.* High overhead are wind-driven rags of clouds passing rapidly across the moon's winking face.

*

Why are you taking them so far away, it's a four-hour drive for me he'd complained bitterly. Her former husband yet not the children's former father. For he would always be their father, so long as he, and they, lived.

*

Only after the labor of birth, only after you've come home to your own private quarters bearing the precious gift of your baby, only then in the abrupt quiet and solitude of ceiling, walls, floor does the realization pierce you like a knifeblade *I am responsible for keeping it alive.*

*

Alone she runs along darkened Spruce Street past dim shapes of houses so similar to her own glimpsed in the corner of her eye they might be interchangeable, identical. It's October, it's night and gusty in chill liquidy moonlight and her ponytail lifts and falls between her shoulder blades as she runs, swinging her slender-muscled arms she runs, her fists lightly clenched, her feet flying lightly touching the pavement and springing away, and on. And on. No one observing in the insomniac night she has claimed at last as her own. *How happy I am, how free I am, no one knows where I am, who I am no one knows.* Holly and Mark are safe in their beds in their snug rooms she, the mother, has provided for them. The other nights she'd slipped away to run they'd slept undisturbed, not knowing she was gone, suspecting nothing. *Where's the harm?*—all the doors and windows of the house are locked, her car is parked as usual beneath the car port so it would appear she's home; no intruder would dare try to enter.

Here in Edgewater, New Jersey. Where nothing has happened for a hundred years. Where nothing will happen, to alarm. *The town that time forgot: Edgewater, New Jersey.* As the real estate agent said with a wink.

*

Why can't I speak with my children without you monitoring our conversations on the phone he'd asked in a voice of aggrieved dignity, his scientist-voice by which as a young wife she'd been intimidated but now empowered by distance she'd said quietly, just slightly provocatively *Of course when you're with them, when they're in your custody no one is monitoring you, but when they're in my custody, beneath my roof, the telephone too is beneath my roof, it's my responsibility isn't it?* Unspoken between them were the bitter accusations she'd made and he'd denied, reiterated through their lawyers like echoes that reverberated without end. He said, making an effort to disguise his deep rage at her *Judith please, it isn't necessary for us to hate each other just because we no longer love each other* and she'd laughed stung, as if the man's words possessed still the capacity for hurt, she laughed *Why not?* and he said *Judith? What? I didn't hear* and she said *You heard me clearly enough, Gabriel* then rethought her position for of course she feared him, she feared him revenging himself upon her through the children, quickly relenting *Of course we don't hate each other, we're civilized adults aren't we?*

Still she continues to listen on the telephone extension when her ex-husband speaks with the children. Never can she imagine a time, her mind at ease, she will not be compelled to listen.

It isn't just their love, their allegiance he wants but their souls. In all broken marriages it is the children's souls that are contested.

For though the man is her ex-husband and no longer shares her bed, he remains the children's father. DNA testing would confirm what she understands to be fact, fate. Out of what unfathomable void, what far-flung careening galaxies. Male seed, female egg. Brainless, eyeless. So simple! And the two children innocently linking them, so long as they both live.

*

Running in the night in the insomniac night she thinks of none of this. Truly.

*

In the night in the wind-buffeted insomniac night she runs. At the corner of Spruce and Highgate passing the First Presbyterian Church of Edgewater, next morning at 10 a.m. she will take Holly and Mark to the Sunday school class in the basement, she'll eagerly attend services upstairs with the mostly retired, predominantly middle-aged and elderly congregation, only a scattering of women and fewer men her own age, she will make an effort to concentrate, to listen to Reverend Heideman's drowsy sermon, she will hope to feel her heart expand with Christian compassion and elation as she sings from the hymnal glancing covertly right and left, hopefully *You see?—I am one of you, no different from any of you.* By night, however, the church that is a historic Edgewater landmark, built 1841 of fieldstone and granite, appears scarcely recognizable. By wind-buffeted moonlight an awkwardly shaped mound of rubble, an untidy ruin beyond straggly trees, slovenly shrubs. What has happened to the church? Has she turned onto the wrong street, confused in the darkness? But no: she recognizes the minister's house adjoining the church, she has visited that house but it too appears changed, squat and misshapen as if its foundation has partly collapsed. Running in the street in the dark she can't slow to look more closely, fear touches her heart and she keeps her gaze resolutely ahead, telling herself it's imagination merely, her fevered imagination, what had her smug pathologist husband predicted for her—*nervous collapse, dissolution of personality*—if she'd persisted in filing for divorce, demanding primary custody of Holly and Mark. But she'd defied him, proven him wrong. How wrong, he has fully to learn.

From Highgate she turns abruptly onto South Main Street, altering her route. She's shaken, confused. Running now past streetlamps that burn with a faint yellow-tinctured light. Past the Edgewater library past the fire station past the township office—all darkened. The pharmacy, the dry cleaner's, the barber shop—darkened. Yet there is Gino's Pizzeria which usually closes by 9 p.m. weekdays, 11 p.m. weekends, still open; a few doors away, Edgewater Video is open too, in fact glaring with light. Patrons in both places are mostly teenagers, she sees. High school kids, here and there a familiar face—a girl named Sandy who'd babysat for her, a tall curly-haired boy named Todd who's mowed her lawn. But most of the kids are strangers, hanging about on the sidewalk, idly smoking, drinking from cans, laughing raucously. She's surprised, disapproving—isn't Edgewater supposed to be a quiet village, not a gathering place for rowdy adolescents? She crosses the street not wanting to pass too close to them but sees nonetheless, to her discomfort, that several of the loutish long-haired boys are staring at her, grinning—as if they know her?—do they know *her*?—and on the steps of the video rental is a bevy of girls, startlingly young girls, in tank tops and jeans as if it's a summer night not a chill October night, the girls slyly cut their eyes at her, too, ducking and giggling, for they're passing what appears to be a joint among them, one of them a slender pale-blond child so resembling Holly that Holly's mother blinks in astonishment, immediate denial *No: impossible* without hesitating for an instant in her running, head turned resolutely away and eyes fixed ahead, a sick trembling inside her *But no: impossible* and she does not glance back, she's eager to be gone from Main Street which has been a mistake on a Saturday night and one she won't repeat.

Except: she'd jogged through downtown Edgewater last weekend, hadn't she, at midnight, it was deserted as a ghost town.

Except: the child wasn't Holly, at least eleven, twelve years old hardly an eight-year-old, *calm down you're imagining things, just calm down* the pathologist-husband's voice admonishes not unkindly. In fact Judith had scarcely glimpsed the girl's face only the silky pale-gold hair, so lovely, so like Holly's. Of the very hue her own had been, at that age.

*

The pathologist, the dissector. Amateur photographer. Fussy with his cameras, please don't touch my cameras. Posing the children, developing his own prints, a perfectionist. How many portraits of her, the attractive smiling young wife so long as she was young. *Why did you ever love me if you can't love me now?* In such awe of him when first they'd met, she an undergraduate nineteen years old dismayed by organic chemistry and he her section instructor, Gabriel, the very name Gabriel, great-winged angel bearer of celestial wisdom *Gabriel.* Six years older than Judith but of another generation, in his presence she'd felt her personality so undefined, anxious simply dissolve like vapor felt her heart beat calmly as if with his magician's fingers he'd reached into her rib cage to cup it. *But this isn't love, this is a place you've walled me up inside, and the children please don't claim this is love.* The past several years he'd taken up videotaping as a hobby, mostly of the children of course, something fanatic in his zeal to record, record, record. By then she'd ceased loving him but not fearing him. Yet daring to object to the videotaping, Holly's seventh birthday and the child was over-excited, feverish with Daddy's attention, exactitude, *Don't you believe anything is real unless you've measured it and recorded it?* and he'd retorted as if she'd asked an idiotic question at the end of a lecture *Every attribute of a thing increases its reality, every truth we can discover about a thing defines it more precisely* and she smiled angrily *Are our children things? Are we things?* and he said *We share "thingness" with all matter, animate or inanimate. Of what do you imagine we're composed, Judith, except matter? The difference between us is that you seem to be ashamed of such facts while I, a scientist, consider them profound.* She laughed, stung. *Profound!*—the fury in the man's face shut like a fist, steely eyes behind the lenses of his glasses narrowed in contempt of her, a mere woman: female body: unexpectedly resistant to his instruments of dissection. She said stammering *It's dead matter you love! Not living people it's dead matter you love!* Lashing out at him where he stood watching her the children hushed, in the next room surely listening. How she hated losing control, a woman losing control to a man as if surrendering her very body's heat to his as in his authority he sucked it from her like that species of giant water spider sucking life from frogs anesthetized by spider venom. *It's deadness you love! Where nothing changes, everythingisfixed!*—shestammerednotknowingwhatshesaidaswithashowofpatience Gabrielblewhisnose,leftnostrilfirst,thentheright,fastidiouslythenrefoldingthehandkerchieftoreturntohispocket. Hesaid *There'swhereyou'remistaken,Judith* calmly, with professorial logic *"Dead matter"* is not permanent, it changes as much as, or more than, "life matter." Its chemicals break down, it decomposes, as fascinating a process as "composing," I assure you—if you aren't blinded by convention, or your own narrow womanly perspective.

Yet she'd won. In the end, the woman won. Taking the children from the man who'd been her husband for nearly ten years. Going into debt for thousands of dollars borrowing to pay her lawyer convinced she was right; would be vindicated. Gabriel had fought her yet principled as he was, adamant in egoism, he had been forced to admit in court that his work schedule and his work addiction made it unlikely he'd be able to spend as many hours weekly with the children as she spent with them even with her commuting and her work. The judge, a black woman, had openly sympathized with the mother in this instance, there'd been a revolution in certain quarters regarding single mothers who worked, Judith had won, or nearly—she had not complete custody of the children, of course, the father had visitation rights, and had expressed satisfaction with the judgment. Not to the judge nor to the lawyers but in an undertone to Judith smiling, shrugging *Well!—the children will be for my older years, then. I have plenty of time in which to win them.*

*

Beyond the estuary of the shallow Millstone River, smelling faintly of garbage rumored to be dumped by night, a harsher undercurrent of chemicals from factories many miles upstream, Judith is running now on the Shore Road, the third side of the rectangle. On previous nights this mile-long stretch beside the ocean has been the high point, the most pleasurable part of her run, despite the perpetual wind; tonight, already she's beginning to tire, her breath has lost its rhythm, there's a twinge of pain in her left knee. The Shore Road is gravel and sand and mud, she can't seem to find solid ground running in patches of darkness as, with a faint sound of jeering laughter, shreds of clouds race across the moon. Non-residents of Edgewater, city people, own most of the property on this road, summer "cottages" large as houses, or mansions; all are shut for the season. Yet Judith sees, or thinks she sees, lights burning here and there, hears voices, outbursts of laughter. Drunken parties, at this time of year? She ignores such distractions, concentrates on her running, her breathing, her control.

In the night in the insomniac night where sudden shadows loom gigantic and in the next instant, vanish, much is exaggerated, Judith knows.

Thinking *Not Holly, don't be ridiculous. Not my daughter not now not ever.*

AWAKE!

In the corner of her eye seeing, not seeing. What is it?—a vehicle parked in the dunes. Headlights off. On a beach trail amid tall rushes, whipped by the wind. She refuses to acknowledge it, will not be alarmed. The vehicle might be abandoned; if anyone is in it, probably they're teenagers, lovers aroused by moonlight; caught up in passion, sexual need, like water swirling deliriously down a drain; unaware of their surroundings, certainly of a lone woman jogging along the Shore Road. If the vehicle is a rusty lead-colored van, its sides painted over so the original words, like cuneiform, are indecipherable, she does not see. *Don't be ridiculous. Look straight ahead, mind your own business.* Yet forced to recall how early that morning the telephone had rung and she'd lifted the receiver to silence—a human, palpable silence. Whispering *Gabriel? Is that you?* Seeing her former husband's face: glinting eyeglasses, stubborn set of the jaw. *Gabriel? Please don't do this. I'm going to hang up now.* He wasn't to pick up the children until a week from Friday, he wouldn't violate that agreement—would he? A man of his professional stature and reputation would not risk any sort of embarrassing domestic scandal—would he? But that afternoon, a disturbing incident she'd since forgotten, odd she'd forgotten it for it had infuriated her at the time: she'd brought Mark to the Edgewater library for a children's reading hour and afterward crossing the street to her car, Mark's moist fingers securely in hers, she'd glanced up to see him—*him*: the walnut-dark man: and in that instant the realization came to her *Of course!*—*he's an emissary of Gabriel's.* A spy, a threat. A reminder. A warning. She wanted to shout *Leave us alone! You have no right, I'll call the police! I know who you are.* But of course she said nothing, dared say nothing. Casting the gnomish creature a scathing look as he seemed almost to be preening himself, displaying himself, only a few yards from the rear of her car, one foot up on a sidewalk bench as he drank from a can—slowly, sensuously, even as his shiny eyes raked over her with a look of blatant sexual assessment. He wore teenaged apparel as if in mockery of his age which was not young, Judith's own age at least—bleached cut-off jeans ragged to his muscular thighs, one of those ugly mustard-yellow sweatshirts with WETLANDS SUCK in black script. Judith flinched at his scrutiny, tugging at Mark who stared at the man, unpredictable Mark lifting a hand to wave at him, at a malevolent stranger, in that way her younger child had of abrupt indiscriminate friendliness: *Hi!*

Judith plunged away with him, breathless into the car fumbling to jam the key into the ignition, slapping at her protesting son scolding *Bad! Bad! Haven't I told you never to—never to so much as look strangers!*

210

The memory returns to her now, vivid and jarring. It isn't an exaggeration to worry that the walnut-dark man has driven the van out here to await her, knowing her itinerary—is it? *Don't think, don't think such things. He will have triumphed if you do.* She runs by, runs past. Bold, indifferent. Seeing how by moonlight the beach appears coarse and riddled as a lunar landscape, crevices and debris and sunken patches like quicksand and a lacy reeking mantel of long-tendrilled glistening things that must be jellyfish, a terrible invasion of jellyfish along the Jersey coast, appalling, mysterious. Such mass deaths, desolation: the purposelessness of nature: a frenzy of reproduction, crazed life brought into being but fleetingly, much of it turned immediately back to pulp, protoplasm. *What is the point of it?* Judith had more than once inquired of her husband, bemused, yet disturbed, at similar anomalies in nature in the early days of her marriage to a man she'd believed to be a man of wisdom as well as merely of facts. And Gabriel had said, not unkindly *Judith, questions about the "point" of things in nature suggest wishful thinking on the part of the questioner.* And Judith said, with a despairing little laugh *But can't there be a point, a purpose, in nature, as well as just a "wish" in the questioner?* And Gabriel laughed, kissed her as he might have kissed a charmingly impertinent child.

Yes, those shapes are jellyfish, or their remains. Luminous by moonlight as if somehow still alive. And here and there amid tangled debris a glisten of dead fish, animal carcasses, bleached detached bones. Though Judith knows these things aren't human in any way human merely creaturely remains cast up by the waves she has to look quickly away. When first she'd brought her excited children to hike along the Edgewater shore the previous spring, at the time she'd signed the lease for the house, the state had just completed a massive clean-up after a devastating winter, and the shoreline had been beautiful in its modest way, hospitable for wading if not for swimming; by late summer, pollution and hurricane damage had altered it considerably. Erosion, inches each year, how many inches the entire Atlantic seacoast. Inexorable, inevitable. As life sucks at life, building up in one place even as another is depleted, exhausted. *I have plenty of time in which to win.*

*

The van's motor has started, the headlights have been switched on. Judith tries not to panic hearing the vehicle bounce over the dunes and down onto the road; headed in her direction; approaching her but not passing; keeping a distance of perhaps thirty feet; teasing? taunting? or out of courtesy not wanting to pass too close to her? She's running at the very edge of the road, refuses to run in the ditch. Refuses to break suddenly and run onto someone's property, into a marshy field, hide in underbrush like a hunted animal, try to escape her pursuer. Suddenly she's covered in sticky sweat, she can smell herself; her hair loose, slipped from the ponytail and whipping in the wind. *Why! why had she come out to this lonely place,* at such a time of night? Leaving her sleeping children behind, what could she have been thinking of? *Any punishment, you know you'll deserve.* The van's brash bright glaring headlights sweep onto her exposing her straining body as in an X-ray.

But Judith manages to run as before, or nearly. Trying not to limp so the driver of the van won't know there is anything wrong. As if she isn't frightened either. As if this—the loneliness, the late hour, the teasing pursuit—is nothing remarkable, nothing she can't handle. And finally at the intersection of the road with a narrower road leading inland the driver of the van speeds up to pass her and she swallows hard feeling a thrill of terror she'll be struck, killed instantly as the motor's roaring grows louder and louder and she can't stop herself stumbling into a ditch screaming as with a blare of its horn and derisive male laughter the van rushes past.

Leaving her sobbing in relief, cringing in pain at the side of the road, her ankle twisted.

*

Please don't make me hate you, hatred is exhausting.
A woman does not exult in hating: not like a man.
Wish only that he. Not death exactly, but.
Yes if he'd disappear! Simply—cease to exist.

Several times since moving to Edgewater she has had the dream and it leaves her faint with shame, excitement. In a foreign country, India perhaps, somewhere she has never visited, he has died—attending one of his science conferences, all expenses paid. But he has died, is dead. Is vanished. It seems that the funeral (funeral pyre? cremation?) has already been held, and the burial. No need for her and the children to attend. The body has been cleanly disposed of, the man himself erased. *Ashes, dust. Bones rising from the earth as plumes of powdery smoke.*

Of course the children would grieve for their father, for a while; and then forget. As children do. Healthy children.

*

Except. That incident of several weeks ago, alone and possibly she'd been drinking (only wine, only a few glasses) and she'd fallen asleep on the sofa anxious, headachy in sleep awaiting the children's safe return, Sunday promptly by 8 p.m. he must return her children to the door of the rented house like clockwork and he and she exchange civil words like the civil, civilized adults they are but afterward, at bedtime, she smelled—what?—ether?—sweet sickish odor in their hair and on their clothes, no mistaking it. Suddenly frantic questioning the little girl *Holly what did he do to you? Oh God, Holly—your father—what did he do to you and Mark?* tearing at their clothes to examine them, their small quivering naked bodies, until Holly began to cry pushing at her mother's hands and Mark ran from her crying and she was left dull-eyed squatting on her heels her hair in her face realizing it must have been a dream. Not the dream of his death but that other so ugly she could only barely recall it by day. Confusing a dream with—whatever this is surrounding us.

*

Once upon a time, a very special time, there was a mommy and a little girl and a little joy who. Nothing not happy, a happy surprise. In the night in the insomniac night breathless and limping returning at last to the stone-and-stucco bungalow on a street whose name she has forgotten in a state of dread and guilt for it's very late— by her watch 2:20 a.m.—much later than she'd intended to stay out. And seeing with a shock of horror a light burning in a window at the rear of the house. One of the children's rooms: Mark's. She hurries panting to the window to peer inside, pushing away brambles, unable to see anything at first because the venetian blind is shut but she hears sounds, children's squeals, a man's deep teasing-cajoling voice, it's Gabriel? Gabriel with the children? taking advantage of her absence, her carelessness? Judith leans against the window managing to catch a glimpse through the blind's slats of pale naked squirming flesh, child-flesh, a man's straining back, video camera in his hands, she screams *No! Stop!* bringing her fist against the window pounding through the screen until the glass cracks then she's at the back door *but the door is locked!* fumbling with her key the key in her fingers slippery with sweat but she manages to unlock the door, he'd forgotten to double-bolt it from inside, she's rushing through the darkened house as the floor tilts drunkenly beneath her as in an earthquake, she slams open the door to Mark's room crying *No! Stop! I'll kill you!* but to her amazement Mark is alone curled beneath the covers of his bed, only the Mother Goose lamp on the floor emits its gentle light and she switches on the overhead light furious and baffled seeing that the man is gone, the father has escaped, with a start the child wakes and opens his eyes blinking in a pretense of surprise and alarm as his mother shakes him *Where is he? what have you been doing together? I saw you! I saw you!* shaking the child's thin shoulders, hugging him tight against her, she's

AWAKE!

weeping angrily, sees his pajamas are back on, hurriedly Gabriel must have dressed their son and of course the child will protect the father as always, they are in league against her. She drags Mark into Holly's room again slams open the door, fumbles to switch on the overhead light seeing her daughter in a pretense of white-faced wide-eyed terror sitting up in bed, clutching the quilt to her chin *Mommy? Mommy what's wrong?* as Judith tears the quilt from her believing the little girl naked but in fact Holly too is wearing her pajamas, exactly as Judith had left her hours before which upsets and infuriates Judith to know that the father and the children have plotted together so shrewdly! so capably! as if not for the first time. She has pushed Mark onto Holly's bed, she has seized both struggling children in her arms, she will protect them, she has driven their father away, always it will be within her power, the mother's power, to drive the father away weeping hot bitter tears *Thank God! Thank God! You're safe!*—knowing one day the hysterical children would realize what it was, their mother had saved them from.

DEAD SLEEP
LYNNE TILLMAN

He told himself not to be afraid of death. He told himself it would be like sleep, eternal and mindless, a pallid time without time and dreams. He told himself he hadn't known he wasn't alive when he wasn't, so death would simply come and carry him from sleep to sleep, and he'd never know life's absence or lost presence. It would be, he told himself, as if he'd never been born.

But ever since he was a child and comforted himself with these morbid thoughts, the relationship between nightly unconsciousness and the absolute end of consciousness undid him. He feared falling asleep because he might, he explained to his mother, wake up dead. He feared being cold and begged his father to promise to bury him in a coffin with a blanket and pillow. A bemused, somewhat anxious father acceded to his son's wishes. But his father was now dead and his mother ill; he was alone. There was no one he could trust to honor a childish request, to sit by his bed, hold his hand, or watch him as he drifted off.

No one could ever know where siren sleep would lead. Each night the man fought physiology's demands, pummeled his pillow, rose from his tormented bed, propped himself, like a puppet, at the window, wrote in his journal, an insomniac's bible, then returned, defeated, to his place of distress. On rare occasions sleep overwhelmed him, and he succumbed to its caresses as he might a lover he couldn't satisfy. During the day sleeplessness disoriented him. He forced himself to work, and his success as a criminal lawyer startled especially him. But his lovers abandoned him. After sex he was restless, and though each woman cajoled and reassured him, his absorbing obsession took over and consumed him. They were never part of it. Finally he resorted to sleeping pills whose chemical ministrations he hadn't wanted before—another erratic element in a tempestuous life. But without sleep he couldn't control his days, either. He had felt compelled to supplicate the demon god of night. The pills wore down his resistance; chemicals lit up his brain in strangely glowing neon patterns. During the first narcotized sleep, blood streamed in front of his eyes, and, upon waking, he imagined he'd gone to the theater and watched a horror movie. Still, a horrible vision was preferable to none.

AWAKE!

Time passed irrevocably. The insolent pills by the side of his bed glowed at him. They had him now. Sleep could be his only through their agency. He had none. With an urgency and devotion new to him, he submitted and swallowed and gave himself over to the brightly colored capsules. Slowly he started to love sleep, love it too much, like a slave who actually adored his master. He had let sleep defeat him, he told himself, it had needed help. But, in its silky arms, he didn't care. Soon he didn't want to wake up. His long-playing dreams escorted him to places he would never have gone awake. He cavorted, unsexed and oversexed, with women and men, delighted in gore, and turned sullen and violent like an unexpected storm. He was an assassin, he was put to death and yet remained alive. He played the executioner who occasionally refused to push the button or wield the axe. Sometimes he quietly watched the dead, who now only looked asleep. Sweet, thick sleep devoured him. He wanted it all the time, he could never get enough. Sleep before time, sleep before mother and father, sleep before love, sleep before discontent. Sleep a nation, a homeland, where his voice was his, not his, and everybody's. Sleep, heavy and brilliant and immense in its singular, lonely, fantastic universe, was preferable to every sensation the other existence extended to him.

The man stopped fearing death. He was free. He swallowed more and more pills. He lost all sense of conscious life, its happy and sad surprises, and when he woke up dead, he did not, of course, know it.

FRIDAY

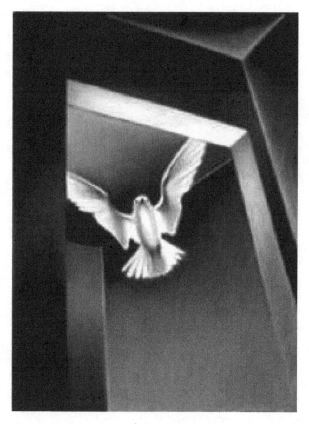

Latent

DREAMS DEFERRED
A. ROGER EKIRCH

"Bed is a medicine," instructs an Italian proverb. Increasingly, Americans are inverting that counsel by ingesting sleeping pills to speed their slumber.

With complaints of insomnia mounting and marketing by drug companies becoming ever more ubiquitous, we are turning in increasing numbers to drugs like Ambien and Lunesta. According to a recent report from the research company IMS Health, pharmacists in the United States filled some 42 million prescriptions for sleeping pills last year, a rise of nearly 60 percent since 2000.

Are we running too quickly to the medicine cabinet? Or is insomnia genuinely reaching epidemic proportions, a consequence perhaps of the frenetic pace of modern life?

In all likelihood, we have never slept so soundly. Yes, the length of a single night's sleep has decreased over the years (upward of 30 percent of adults average six or fewer hours), but the quality of our sleep has improved significantly. And quality, not quantity, sleep researchers tell us, is more important to feeling well rested.

This is not to minimize the torment of insomnia over the course of a restless night. But for most of us, slumber is reasonably tranquil—especially when compared to what passed for a night's rest before the modern era. Despite nostalgic notions about sleep in past centuries, threats to peaceful slumber lurked everywhere, from lice and noxious chamber pots to tempestuous weather.

Worst in this pre-penicillin age was sickness, especially such respiratory tract illnesses as influenza, pulmonary tuberculosis and asthma, all aggravated by bedding rife with mites. One 18th-century diarist recounts that asthma forced her husband to sleep in a chair for months, with "watchers" required to hold his head upright. Among the laboring poor, whose living conditions were horrendous, sleep deprivation was probably chronic, prompting many to nap at midday, much to the annoyance of their masters.

As if these maladies were not enough, we now also know that pre-industrial families commonly experienced a "broken" pattern of sleep, though few contemporaries regarded it in a pejorative light. Until the modern age, most households had two distinct intervals of slumber, known as "first" and "second" sleep, bridged by an hour or more of quiet wakefulness. Usually, people would retire between 9 and 10 o'clock only to stir past midnight to smoke a pipe, brew a tub of ale or even converse with a neighbor.

Others remained in bed to pray or make love. This time after the first sleep was praised as uniquely suited for sexual intimacy; rested couples have "more enjoyment" and "do it better," as one 16th-century French doctor wrote. Often, people might simply have lain in bed ruminating on the meaning of a fresh dream, thereby permitting the conscious mind a window onto the human psyche that remains shuttered for those in the modern day too quick to awake and arise.

The principal explanation for this enigmatic pattern of slumber probably lies in the nocturnal darkness that enveloped pre-industrial households—in short, the absence of artificial lighting. There is a growing consensus on the impact of modern lighting on sleep. The Harvard chronobiologist Charles A. Czeisler has aptly likened lighting to a drug in its physiological effects, producing, among other changes, altered levels of melatonin, the brain hormone that helps to regulate our circadian clock.

In fact, during clinical experiments at the National Institute of Mental Health, human subjects deprived of light at night for weeks at a time exhibited a segmented pattern of sleep closely resembling that related in historical sources (as well as that still exhibited by many wild mammals). The subjects also experienced, during intervals of wakefulness, measurably higher levels of prolactin, the hormone that allows hens to sit happily upon their eggs for long periods.

These elevations of prolactin reinforce historical descriptions of complacent feelings at "first waking" and, back then, probably helped calm people's worries about the night's perils. Prolactin is also what differentiates segmented sleep, with its interval of "non-anxious wakefulness" that nearly resembles a meditative state, from the tossing-and-turning insomnia we medicate against. "Let the end of thy first sleep raise thee from thy repose: then hath the body the best temper; then hath thy soul the least encumbrance," wrote the moralist Francis Quarles.

Remarkably, then, our pattern of consolidated sleep has been a relatively recent development, another product of the industrial age, while segmented sleep was long the natural form of our slumber, having a provenance as old as humankind (Homer even invoked the term "first sleep" in The Odyssey, Book 4). For experts like Dr. Thomas Wehr, who conducted the experiments at the National Institute of Mental Health, this helps to explain common sleep disorders, some of which may be nothing more than sleep's older, primal pattern trying to reassert itself—"breaking through," as Dr. Wehr has put it, into today's "artificial world."

That, of course, remains to be seen. In the meantime, rather than resort to excessive medication, Americans might benefit from a more realistic attitude toward their slumber. Probably we expect too much. Rarely in the past was human slumber so seamless. We might, on occasion, even choose to emulate our ancestors, for whom the dead of night, rather than being a source of dread, often afforded a welcome refuge from the regimen of daily life.

MEDICINE OF BED RIGHT AWAY
Matthew Roher

Broken or dreaming, I lay there talking
with my mouth closed, I could see them, they weren't
clawing me in sleep. A fire in my ears
smells like bitter tea. My wife fitfully
crashed upon the shore. I wonder if
the whole house shuddered & what bitter sickness
means but it sounds pretty. Medicine
of bed right away & work towards that end.
My teeth held themselves all night like a beast's
to myself when I died. I must get out
unseasonably warm & sick, no sleep.
That word you always say. I know that
I will be reassuring company

to my friends who aren't there.

FROM THE INSOMNIA DRAWINGS
LOUISE BOURGEOIS

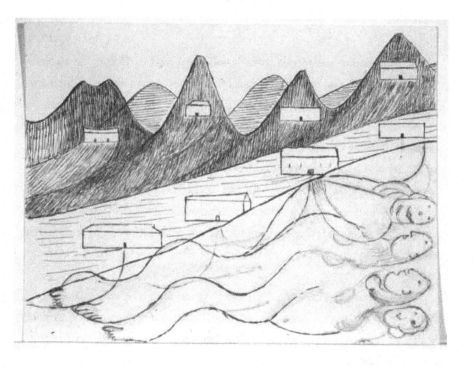

The Insomnia Drawings (detail), 1994-1995
220 mixed media works on paper of varying dimensions
Daros Collection, courtesy Cheim & Read, New York
Photo: Christopher Burke

THE MOST HORRIFIC EIGHT HOURS OF ANYBODY'S LIFE WHO EVER EXISTED ON THE PLANET, BAR NONE, EXCEPT FOR PERHAPS MAYBE, BUT ONLY MAYBE NOW, JESUS

Steve Brykman

When I read in the Herald that Mass General was conducting an insomnia study, it sounded like an easy thing to pull off. Easier even than the generalized anxiety disorder trials I'd undergone last month, and twice as profitable. Better yet, this one wouldn't involve any drugs. All I had to do was let them wire my brain up to a bunch of machines, then lie down for a couple nights, as sleeplessly as I could. It was the wrong thing to do. I know that now. But I've done a lot of wrong things in my life more wrong than this one, and besides, four hundred bucks is four hundred bucks.

The key to being a successful test subject is in the details. So I went online and did my homework, studied up on symptoms, got the lingo down. I found some real doozies, polysomnogram being my favorite. I'd be sure to work that one in somewhere.

The secretary was a permed and dyed woman with crooked but kindly eyes. She spoke to me in a hypnotic near-whisper, as though trying to put me to sleep right there in the waiting-room. Which she nearly did. It's the way we talk to someone terminal, afraid our words alone may be enough to do them in.

Then she handed me a clipboard and, guilt-ridden, asked that I please fill it out:

Q: Do you have difficulty falling or staying asleep?
A: YES and/or YES

Q: Do you awaken from sleep not feeling rested?
A: Frequently I wonder if I've woken up at all.

Q: How often do you awaken at night?
A: Anywhere from 2 to 87 times.

Q: Do you drink much coffee?
A: Only when awake.

Q: Do you have any excessive stress or anxiety?
A: I wouldn't say it's excessive, but after my dad saw the inside
   of my medicine cabinet, he bought a thousand shares of Merck.
   Badump-bum.

Q: What do you do during the few hours before you go to bed?
A: Brood, fret, torment myself generally.

Q: Are you often falling asleep?
A: Sometimes even in my dreams.

Q: Do you fall asleep at inappropriate times or places?
A: Once. At my grandfather's funeral. But in my defense, it was a
   very dry ceremony.

Q: Do you have breath-holding spells?
A: Does that include underwater?

Q: Do you have any aches or pains that prevent you from sleeping?
A: If you count psychological scars from early childhood, then yes.

Q: Do you snore?
A: I wouldn't know. I'm asleep at the time.

Thank you very much and don't forget to tip your waitress.

This was not going to be a problem, I assured myself. So maybe I didn't have
chronic insomnia, by definition. So maybe I wasn't what you might call a classic text-

book example. So maybe—truth be told—sleeping is one of the few things I pride myself on and manage to do consistently well. So what? Is that any reason why I shouldn't take part in an insomnia study? Especially in an age when our own FDA is in cahoots with the drug companies? Where deadly side-effects are kept hidden from the hapless public? Why, I'll be checking up on them, making sure their methods are sound. I'm a watchdog for the common man, behaving in accordance with the tenor of the times.

There were any number of things I could keep myself awake over. I've done it a thousand times. My list is extensive. In the "not enough of" category, we have: Cash, Short Term Memory, Time, and Sexual Potency. In the "too much of" category, you'll find: Girth, Pot-Smoking, and Surfing the Net for Free Porn. But the one worry that currently stands head and shoulders above the rest, the one that's been keeping me up for the last couple weeks, is my father, who is at this moment lying in Sinai with a catheter in his crotch, waiting patiently for a quadruple bypass.

*

By the time they got me all wired up, I was already jonesing for a nap. Thankfully, my room had a television and I could watch as much as I wanted. I made up my mind to find the most insipid reality programming offered and embrace it like a Chekhov play until my own reality was but a faded, empty dream. But I also came prepared. I had hatched a backup plan in the event that I found myself drifting off at 3 a.m. No matter what degree of examination they were planning to give me, I felt pretty confident it wasn't going to involve my nuts. So I crushed a bunch of No-Doz into a doll-sized Ziploc and taped it to the underside of my balls. If I got tired I would simply dip a moistened finger in the powder and inconspicuously lick it clean.

Despite the state-of-the-art equipment that surrounded me, monitoring my every electrical impulse (polysomnograms and all), by 8 p.m. the batteries in my remote control were failing. I took it as a bad omen, potentially indicating a downturn in my father's condition. I was unable to change channels and got stuck with Dateline NBC. No big deal. Could be worse. I could have four blocked arteries and a cardiac pump keeping me alive. Stone Phillips was interviewing this fat, balding, older white guy and he's talking about getting sliced up and the pain from the clamps and whatnot and I'm thinking maybe he was attacked by a gang or something until I finally figure out that what happened was that this guy had actually—no bullshit—

woken up in the middle of heart surgery. Apparently, Western anesthetics have little to no effect on him. I don't remember the exact title of the segment, but it may as well have been: *The Most Horrific Eight Hours of Anybody's Life Who Ever Existed on the Planet, Bar None, Except For Perhaps Maybe, But Only Maybe Now, Jesus.* I'm paraphrasing, but the dialogue went something like this:

Anesthetic-Resistant Man: "... when I woke up they had my thorax wide open. I could feel the wind in my chest cavity."

Stone: "That's disgusting."

Anesthetic-Resistant Man: "I could feel them cutting into me, sawing through my breastbone. I started flashing back. For a while there I thought I was in Nam. They kept me locked in solitary for months and tortured me almost on a daily basis. But this surgery thing, man, this was worse."

Stone: "You wanted desperately to speak out ..."

Anasthetic-Resistant-But-Soon-to-be-Filthy-Rich-Off-His-Out-of-Court-Settlement Man: "I couldn't. I couldn't say or do anything. See, part of what the anesthesia does is it totally paralyzes you. Lucky me, huh? I got the paralysis without the pain-killing. They got me in therapy now ..."

I shut off the TV. I couldn't for a second allow myself to entertain the thought of Dad going through something like that. But it was too late. The idea was already bouncing around in my head and it wouldn't leave. It felt like a sign. There were disturbing similarities. My father was also an overweight balding white man who had served in the war. I knew he couldn't handle seeing this show, not on the night before his own bypass with a pump stuck in his vein. He was already nervous enough as it was. Long ago, he'd made a promise to himself never to undergo any sort of heart surgery. Because shortly after his own mother went in for her bypass she became demented, believed Nazis were landing helicopters atop Hebrew Rehab, and shortly thereafter, died. To this day, he blames the doctors.

227

I prayed he was watching the game.

I plunged my finger in my groin and licked off the bitterness.

Ten minutes later, I had the jitters. My concern for my father existed in my mind on a multitude of disturbing levels. Not only was I of course worried for his well-being, I also couldn't help thinking that between us there remained a lot of work to be done. That here I was, lying in a similar bed just a few miles away for no good reason at all except to milk the system for a few hundred bucks when, the last time I saw my father, the best final words he could muster were, "Well, it was nice knowing you." Not exactly the sort of emotionally ground-breaking stuff one would hope for from a man who believed his life might be about to end. There had been no father-son coming to terms, just as it had been with his own father before him. And now, if—God forbid—the unspeakable happened while I was in here jerking around the medical community, then that would be it.

No, staying awake these few nights would not be a problem.

I held a Zoloft pen between my now-shaky fingers, turned over my sleep study instructions and spent much of the night drafting the words I would say to my dad when I walked out of Mass General and caught the T to Sinai. I won't print them here but the general message of the thing was that I loved him and that considering he had lived most of his life without his father in it, I thought he had generally done a pretty decent job and I was proud and thankful to have known him.

When I'd finally finished writing, the sky was just beginning to reveal the earliest iridescence of morning. I peeled the countless sticky pads from my heart and the EKG drew a straight unwavering line. Freed from the adhesion, I felt somehow renewed, as if waking from a sound and restful sleep. Though my eyes had yet to close.

HELLO DAVID AXELROD SUPERSTAR
NICK MONTEMARANO

He stayed awake three days straight before he had to take something. A cup of coffee, no big deal. Not a bad start. Coffee got him through the next day, caffeine pills and energy drinks the next. He was feeling good about his chances until he realized that he wasn't even halfway there. He didn't want to have to start popping bennies this soon, but already he was confused, his speech—he was talking to himself—slurred and nonsensical.

He wasn't really talking to himself; he was talking to the camcorder he had set on its tripod in the living room. One hundred twenty hours of video, so far, of him not sleeping. Of him watching TV and listening to music—he had figured that if he listened to all three hundred fifty or so CDs he owned he would be there, or almost there—and talking on the phone to friends who would put up with his blather. Of him doing pushups and sit-ups and jumping jacks and eating bowl after bowl of cereal and ice cream and anything else sugary he had in his apartment. Of him closing his eyes only to rest them, always making sure to continue speaking to prove that he had not fallen asleep, *I am closing my eyes to rest them but I am not sleeping as evidenced by my talking to you right now.* And he could not help imagining this video becoming famous, or at least a kind of cult classic. He couldn't tell if such fantasies were realistic or embarrassing because he could barely recall his own name after day six, and he had promised himself that he would not call Stella, his ex, no matter what, but on day seven he called her at home—he was that loopy—and asked her if she would come over and sit with him for the remaining five days, and when she said no, he was crazy, she had a life, a husband, a three-month-old son, he tried to entice her by telling her she would be part of the film he was making. People will see you, he told her. You'll be famous, he said—a line he would cringe upon hearing when it was all over and he watched the video.

Better to do this alone, he decided. It would be more authentic that way. Randy Gardner had had help (his sister held ice on his back and neck during days ten and eleven; his friend took him for a ride in his convertible with the top down; he had a doctor with him, for God's sake!), but he, David Axelrod—whose name would replace Randy Gardner's, whose name sounded like the name of a famous person, his college drama teacher once told him—*he* wouldn't need help.

Except coffee and caffeine pills and hourly cans of ROCKSTAR and CRUNK!!!, and now, on day eight, bennies. A pill-popping neighborhood acquaintance had given them to him—a gesture of good luck—when David had been bragging about what he hadn't done yet. That was something Stella used to say about him—that he was all talk, that he was a planner, not a doer. She had called him cold and selfish and immature—nice things, too, though he chose not to remember those—but the worst she said of him was that he was lazy and scared of following through, a starter but not a finisher, and sometimes, not even a starter.

By the end of day eight he was having fun—genuine fall-on-the-floor-laughing fun—listening to himself speak. God, he may as well have been speaking Chinese. It sounded as if his lips had frozen, or as if he'd had a stroke. He laughed and laughed and was certain that everything he said into the camera—understandable or not—was profound. He imagined stoned college kids watching his video and inventing a new language based on the words his mouth now seemed to be making up. He was having so much fun that he didn't understand what the big deal was; why such a fuss over staying awake eleven days? Why such a big deal over Randy Gardner, who had been seventeen years old in 1964, when he broke the record, ten years younger than David was now? Even Stella knew who Randy Gardner was, and long before David had become obsessed—not obsessed, but *determined*, he would say—with breaking his record. There was an all-girl punk rock band in Japan called Hello Randy Gardner Superstar, and Stella had a few of their albums. She even took David to see them once, in the East Village, on New Year's Eve. Three tiny Japanese women wearing black leather platform boots that came up over their knees, their hair dyed bright red, arms covered in tattoos, noses and lips and eyebrows and who knew what else pierced, and the sounds that came out of their mouths! Screams, really. Shrieks. David was certain one of them was snarling at him dominatrix-like. He felt somewhat out of place at the show—he was wearing a ski jacket, a winter hat with pompom, and brown duck boots his mother had bought him for Christmas—but he had seen photos of Randy Gardner, and *he* wasn't what David would call cool, not when he was seventeen, and not now at almost sixty years old. Certainly not cool enough to have a band of swearing, boot-stomping, guitar-smashing, stage-diving Japanese women named after him, his name on the drums in large black letters, his name tattooed—David saw when he went on the band's web site—on each member's ass!

He was not the kind of person who wanted to be famous. Not famous-famous. Not really. He didn't want to become some kind of Mark David Chapman by going out and shooting a rock star. But *this* he could do. And it wasn't that he expected a rock band to name themselves after him, but what would Hello Randy Gardner Superstar think of Randy Gardner when Randy Gardner didn't even hold the god-damn stupid record anymore for staying awake the longest? What would Stella and Stella's husband and Stella's ten-month-old son think? Not that a baby could think anything about anything. His thinking—he was now closing in on the end of day nine, and was out of cereal and ice cream and all sugary food products, including sugar itself, which he had been eating by the handful, and was out of ROCKSTAR and CRUNK!!!, and did not trust himself to venture outside, not even to the convenience store on the corner, and besides did not want to walk away from the camera, oth-erwise his cult-classic movie might be criticized for not documenting every hour of the two hundred sixty-five hours he needed to stay awake to break the record, not that he planned to stop at two hundred sixty-five hours, he would go on to three hundred, four hundred, he would go on and on, he would double the fucking record, and he would mail a copy of his movie to Randy Gardner and to each member of Hello Randy Gardner Superstar and to each member of the Hello Randy Gardner Superstar Fan Club and to Stella and her husband and their son, and he would start a web site called Hello David Axelrod Superstar, and he couldn't remember the last time he had changed the tape in the camcorder—his thinking, as would have been clear to him had he been able to think clearly, was a complete mess. One thought rambled into the next. One hour bled into the next, one day into the next—for all he knew, he could have broken the record by now. It was something like what people had described near-death experiences being like. He was hovering above his body but also inside his body. He was in the present moment but also not. His memory, if not his sentences, was clearer than ever. Things he had not remembered in years came back to him. Memories about sleeping or not sleeping. (As a boy, his father long gone, David had nightmares that monsters were going to come down from the attic and kill him [the attic door was in his bedroom, the head of his bed near the door], and until he was four his mother allowed him to sleep in her bed, but after four he had to come up with a new plan, otherwise he would not sleep, would not close his eyes, would not turn out his light, and so he would sneak out of his room and walk as quietly as possible across the hallway and sit at the top of the stairs and watch what his mother was watching on TV, but what his mother often watched were horror movies—vampires, mummies, werewolves, space aliens, killer sharks, killer whales, killer crocodiles, killer spiders, killer bees, killer dogs, killer cars, murderers with ski masks, murderers with hockey masks, child killers with knives for fingers, possessed children, possessed houses, devil worshippers, the devil's baby, dead people come back to life—and by the time his mother turned off the TV and came up to bed, it no longer mattered that she was in the next room, because as soon as he heard her snoring, he may as well have been alone in the world, and he spent the better part of his early childhood awake in bed, waiting for the first glow of sun to lighten his room, so he could finally close his eyes. Ages five through ten: the dream of peeing, the initial release, the satisfaction, then the sudden panic upon realizing that he was in bed and it had happened again, then the attempt to open his dresser quietly so as not to wake his mother, the attempt to change his clothes quietly, the attempt to walk down the hallway to the closet for a clean towel and walk back to his room [the floorboards creaking under his feet], then laying the towel over the wet spot—he had the entire post-bedwetting procedure down to a science—and curling his body on the dry part of the mattress, all the while knowing that his mother knew, of course she did, and during these years he did not sleep over his friends' houses, and when he finally did—he was twelve—he did not actually sleep, but pretended to, getting up every few hours to pee what little was left in his bladder. In college, he wrote SLOPPY DRUNK on his alcoholic roommate's eyelids, one word on each eyelid, and covered his roommate's face and hands with peanut butter, and tied his roommate's wrists and ankles together, and tied his body to the mattress, and recruited a half dozen of his friends to carry the roommate—still on the mattress—outside to the quad, where he woke in the morning. And for this reason, once the roommate went into rehab and quit drinking and started attending meetings, David did not sleep very well, fearing that his roommate, despite his newfound spirituality, wanted revenge, just once: a shaving of the eyebrows, white-out on David's face, something worse David had not yet thought of. To ease his anxiety, David drank more, therefore finding it difficult to stay awake, and he would wake each morning and look in the mirror to see if his roommate had exacted his revenge—if he had shaved half his head or had put his finger in a bucket of water, inducing him to wet his bed [this would have shamed him on several levels, given his history]—but every morning he was fine, a fact that only increased his anxiety the following night, when he would lie in bed, trying to decide if his roommate's rhythmic breathing was the authentic breathing of sleep, or only a ruse to make him let down his guard. By the time David graduated from college he had been sleep-deprived for three plus years, and looked forward to moving back home to New York, where he could finally catch up on sleep, but his body had become so used to getting only a few hours of sleep each night that he wasn't able to get back on a healthy schedule, and for the next few years he saw sleep as a kind of Holy Grail, worshipping it when it did come, resenting it when it did not. [In his present sleep-deprived state, David believed he could see the future, as well as the past: He saw himself at seventy, up every three hours every night to empty his bladder and up for good by four, just like one of those old people he swore and foolishly believed he would never become, an expert in all the lousy TV shows only the truly sleep deprived watch, this one selling you a mop, this one selling you a chair that massages your back, this one selling you new hair, a new nose, a new wife.])

The sun rose on day eleven, only twenty-four hours and one minute from breaking the record. He did not know if he would make it. At some point he had wet his pants, but didn't care. He tried to remember *Invasion of the Body Snatchers*— that could help him now, if nothing else could. He saw it for the first time at the age of six, when he should have been sleeping (it had been one of his mother's favorites), and swore to himself then that if he ever *had* to stay awake, if ever his life depended on it, he could. Forever, if necessary. Just one more naïve idea he'd had as a kid because he didn't know any better. He tried to imagine for the final day that if he fell asleep aliens would replace him with a space pod that looked like him but had no feelings.

Staying awake was becoming painful now, and he could admit at least *some* respect for Randy Gardner. He closed his eyes and kept speaking into the camera, *Hello David Axelrod Superstar, Hello David Axelrod Superstar*, and soon found himself in what he would describe later as a meditative state—relaxed but awake, supremely focused.

By the time he emerged from this trance he was down to the final six hours, enough time to play both of Hello Randy Gardner Superstar's double-albums he had stolen from Stella when he moved out, then play them again, and the final two hours were remarkably easy.

The final minute was anticlimactic.

AWAKE!

The first minute after having broken the record he wasn't sure what to do with himself. He felt like crying—more from exhaustion than from emotion—but couldn't.

His brain was mush, but he had done it, and now, finally, he could sleep.

It was three-fifteen in the morning.

He stacked his two hundred sixty-five hours of tapes, lay on the floor, and closed his eyes. He would sleep for the next two or three days, he decided, and when he woke up he would call a few friends and they would all go out and celebrate.

But there was a buzz.

He thought at first that it was the refrigerator, but it was inside his head. To be expected, he told himself. For God's sake—he had been awake for over eleven days. He was lucky he hadn't gone insane—though if he *had* gone insane, he wasn't sure how he would know. He could deal with the buzzing in his head. No problem. He poured a glass of wine and drank it quickly; he poured another and drank it. The buzz was still there, but now he cared less; it was like the noise a fan made. Soothing.

But an hour later he was still awake.

Fine, he would have to take a sleeping pill. Two, he decided. He wasn't going to mess around.

Being on the floor probably wasn't helping either, so he undressed and got into bed and waited to fall asleep.

Two hours later, he was still waiting.

He didn't want to take any more sleeping pills—not with the two glasses of wine. But what else could he do?

He turned on the TV. Morning news. A kids' show: plastic eyeballs glued to talking hands. A religious program: a tiny woman with a mountainous beehive wig: *Oh happy race of mortals how you have fallen! The light at the end of the tunnel is out until further notice!* He changed the channel: a British man trying to sell him a grill in the shape of a woman's ass, or at least it looked like a woman's ass; meat fat dripped into a pan beneath the grill. The picture on the screen shook as if the program had been filmed during an earthquake. He turned away from the TV and the room shook; he held on to the arms of the couch. Desperate, he flipped once more: as if an answer to a prayer he was too psychotic to have prayed, there was Bob Ross. David couldn't quite see him, but he could hear his voice: unmistakable: a voice like Demerol. Just what he needed. Happy clouds, pine trees, a river bank between snow-covered mountain peaks. He may as well have been blind now—he saw three Bob Ross afros—but his hearing was fine. It didn't even bother him—not much, anyway—when he remembered that Bob Ross was dead, or when he remembered that Stella's new husband's name was Robert and their son's name was Ross.

He lay on the floor, closed his eyes, and waited. A strange but wonderful certainty came over him that his life was going to change, that after he woke from a long sleep, everything would be different, would be better.

Bob Ross said: *We're not committed yet. This is your bravery test. Decide where your little footy hills live. Super. We don't make mistakes, we make happy little accidents.*

When the show ended, he was still awake. Nothing had changed. His name was David Axelrod. He was twenty-seven years old and divorced. He smoked pot once in a while; he drank too much, sometimes. He was smart and liked to read graphic novels; he could draw pretty well; he could talk philosophy at the coffee shop. Most of his friends were married and had kids. He could think of no one he could call at this hour. On the bright side, it was a new day. Eventually, he would fall asleep; he would have to; it would be impossible not to. But for now, with every second that passed, he added, reluctantly, to his own record.

THE WALK
Susan Steinberg

there's the ceiling, the ceiling fan spinning dust, the bed undone underneath, and you're in the bed waking, no, you're always awake when it's this hot, this late, the ceiling fan humming, spinning dust in the dark, then in daylight, its motor a car sound, an idling, a bus sound humming, the fan blades stirring, sweat streaking the bed and the streaks widen, stain, your eyes closed tight, and the room seems outside, open, a bus motor idling, the spin of leaves and rain, a school trip in fall, standing curbside on Lexington near Lexington Market, standing lightheaded in the yellow glare of raincoats, in the hum of the buses, in the squeal on the streets made of glass, they are, said your father, again and again, made of glass, and they glitter, and you need to be inside, shut in the school bus, warm in the bus where your teeth won't chatter, where your skin won't creep, where you're sheltered, clearheaded, and you open your eyes and you're inside, waking, no, always awake, and it's no longer morning and the rain is sweat, the leaves are heat, the yellow raincoats dull to hot air, an undone bed, black shoes in the corner, the black like a pit, like a hole to a cave where you can't hear the fan, where you can't hear it spin, when in Baltimore and in summer, when on Fayette Street, when the phone rings the head throbs, don't answer the phone now, it's time for a walk, when you're ready to stand, you're not ready, get ready,

the pills soften in the throat and the water comes late, warm in the glass, leaving a taste everyone knows as white, aspirin, and white is bitter everyone knows, even your father said, don't chew, swallow, bitter, aspirin, and the pills will kick in, not yet, in an hour, aspirin takes an hour, from noon to one, and you float through the room, slip out of clothing, slip into clothing, under the fan pushing dust, its motor humming, and you hold your black shoes, one in each hand, you float to the window, it's open already, Baltimore shimmering through the window in a haze, Howard Street, Lexington, Calvert, Charles, made of what, said your father, glass, you said, and it glitters in the light, in the white haze of summer, as you drop your black shoes from the window to the walk, and the black shoes will wait for you on the walk, and your hands are free and you can hold air solid, cloudy, on a finger, in a hand, in the crook of an arm, as the phone rings, let it, and the air feels like foam, like sap, squeezed tight in a fist, in the crook of the neck, and below are your shoes curled on the walk, turned to their sides, crooked like what, like pain, no, like laughing, it's funny, and you can't reach the shoes as you live on the top floor and heat rises, everyone knows, even your father said so when you had a fever, when the school bus took you from Lexington Market to in front of your house and you saw the sign for 30th Street, where you ate and slept, where you lived with your mother, your father, where you fell lightheaded to the wet leaves and grass, heavyheaded you had fallen face first to the wet, fainted, said your father as he ran outside, his word riding on a cloud to bring you to, to bring you in, and the heat rose to your head from your wrist and your father said, fever, gave aspirin and ice and covers and you slept, you waked, you slept, you waked,

the glass of water shatters to the walk, to Baltimore, to the shoes on the walk, it was an accident, the glass was wet and slipped, and the water in the glass was warm anyway, and the grass jutting up through cracks in the walk needs the water anyway when there's never rain, not even a spray or mist to break the heat, not even a raincloud, and the water was warm anyway in the glass from the sun throbbing low through the window, and you can hear the sun sounding like a pulse but it's a pulsing in your head, blood pulsing in your wrist, and you can see the blood-pulse jump in one wrist, now the other, as your arms hang limp in the sap, as they hang out the window, and looking at your pulse is looking at your life in slow-motion, how you will always be this, this, this, how your life and the sun are the same pulse-throb throbbing, and your father called you blue-blood from the veins in a wrist, blue-blooded from fainting, he took your pulse, you took an aspirin, don't chew, then covers, ice on your wrist, then quiet, sleep, car sounds in sleep, dreams of fights, of car horns blaring on 30th Street, and you waked in the same place, in the same bed, to your sponge-faced mother, another aspirin, water, Lexington Market still afloat in your head like clouds, like rain, the crabs sideways crawling in wet glass boxes, the birds strung up with blood-soaked rope, the cows staring blankly behind small windows, the buzzing of lights and the smell of food was it, or slaughter you could say today, was it slaughter, the blood, and you wondered of the cows, why everyone laughed in their yellow raincoats and yellow boots, they laughed at what happened behind the small windows, the cows were back there blankly staring, you turned your back to their stares, your front to the scattered raincoats like all the suns burning your eyes when you opened your eyes in Lexington Market, on Lexington Street, on the bus going homeward, on the grass at home, inside with fever to take an aspirin, how you opened your eyes at noon today, in this place, Baltimore, St. Paul Street, Fayette Street, word-named streets, where the buildings shimmer in a sun haze, where the sun seems stuck up there like in glue or in a spread of white plaster, where the shoes on the walk look disfigured, distorted through the heat like shadows of crabs crawling up St. Paul, Fayette, and the heat floats you from the window,

the heat floats you to the darkest room to its darkest corner and you find yourself standing barefoot in the kitchen, you find yourself standing crooked, useless, and it's funny to be barefoot in a kitchen when you almost remember like a dream of what was it when you see your bare feet pressed to the floor and realize there is no one, was there ever, when you were younger with fever, you were sheltered, now you're older with veins in your bare feet, blue blood running through your hot feet, you're older, you're this-old this-old this-old, like twenty like thirty, and the kitchen is dark, the freezer is empty, just ice and cold air, no longer a cave like when your father gave ice, he said, go back to bed you have fever, and, no more Lexington Market for you, and, you can't handle these trips to the market, and you looked in the freezer when you were burning cold-hot and your father said, climb in it's a cave to cool you, and it looked like a cave of frozen dirt, of scratchings on walls of cows and trees, climb in, said your father, but you were already too big and if you could have made yourself smaller, if you could now, if you could crawl inside and curl and sleep like a bear in a cave,

the pills will kick in in an hour, who said an hour, someone said, it's only aspirin, your father said, one hour, he said, you'll be fine by tomorrow, though they don't always kick in, aspirin, and what is the magic of an hour when your head is splitting from no sleep, from heat, what is the magic of timing time when you're always looking to the end, when you always need the other side of an hour, when the other side is sixty minutes away and when you get sixty minutes away you are sixty minutes older and sixty minutes older, when you're lucky, when you're not, when you're lucky, the staircase is soundless, bare feet are silent, thank goodness, when you're throbbing, splitting, and the shoes are waiting there for you on the walk, and the door shuts behind you and you're outside, shoeless, sweating, squinting upward to your window, and it's hard to believe you live behind that window where the fan spins slowly on the ceiling and it seems it should do more, all that life, it should sound more like a bear, less like a motor,

when your father said, go to sleep, you asked of the cows and your father said, sleep, you slept, you heard a motor in your head, a fighting fever-dream, awake in an hour, screaming for your father, the fever unbroken, the dream fading out like a day, almost forgotten, another aspirin, your wrung-out mother saying, swallow,

the phone is still ringing, your father calling from someplace, outside, Florida, but you can't rush inside, it's too hot, you can't rush in to answer, and it's just your father from outside by his car, the motor running, in that place, Florida, saying, hello blue-blood, as he said when you were hazy from fever, he said, come back blue-blood, when you were out there in a fever-dream, burning like summer, when your head was sap, as the sky gets in summer, when your head was a cow's head, blood-rushed and hot, pressed heavy to the wet leaves and grass,

you're standing shoeless near curled shoes and funny to throw your shoes from the window so they could curl in the sun, but the staircase was soundless, goodness, and what right shoes curl from heat, what right shoes crab-crawl on the walk and who said to crash the glass to your shoes, your only glass, but that was an accident, and you're standing shoeless on the shards, an accident, and your foot is bleeding, an accident, really, who can think on a white-hot day in Baltimore in a sun-haze with a throbbing split-up head like with fever, like when your father said, come back, he thought he lost you to fever, isn't this right, it doesn't seem right when there you were in the same bed in the same room in the same house on 30th, waking in an hour to your dried-up mother by the same bed in the same room, just your mother in the room saying, swallow, when your father went, is that right, it wasn't that day was it but another, it wasn't that day was it when he left, don't think it was that day when you were fainted from fever and really can't remember,

AWAKE!

when the fever broke you walked to the kitchen and your mother stood withered, barefoot, looking at the window and it was already funny to be barefoot in a kitchen and you looked in the freezer and it was just a freezer, no longer a cave but dim walls and cold air, how its dim walls and cold air on this word-named street in this same old city on this glaring hazy day today when the sky is so thick and white you can't see clouds floating and you have to ask if anything is still afloat,

it's time, just a walk around the corner, just some air, and you should turn and walk before someone looks from your window, but there's no one, just the phone, but you should walk before someone calls from your window, but really there's no one, you're grown now, you're thirty, you're twenty, you're nineteen eighteen fourteen thirteen, you're nineteen, you're thirty, you should turn and walk before you rush back inside, before you answer the phone, before your father says, hello blue-blood, how's Baltimore blue-blood, can you see the glass streets from your window, can you see Lexington Market from where you live, can you see the crabs sideways crawling in watery cases, can you see the cows' heavy staring and the birds strung up with rope, and he would never say this, but if he did, but he wouldn't, but if he did you would tell him you can see the whole market shimmer from your window and you can smell the crabs, the sand and salt, the blood of the cows, you can hear their blood pulsing when the air is thinner, when the sky is bluer, you can see the window in the market from your window and the cows' heads past the window about to hit the straw floor, the cement floor, and you can see the laughing yellow raincoats, you can see how funny it is to be on the good side of a window and the cows can see you laughing and laughing because you can take it now because you really don't care now because you're grown now, this old, and the cows can see their last see-through and it's you there laughing it up before their heads hit the floor before their time is up,

when the fever broke you walked to the kitchen and your mother stood tired, barefoot, looking out the window, and your father walked in wet-haired, withered, goodness, that day, you remember that day, he'd only been out for a walk,

listen, the phone's still ringing behind your window and listen, the fan's still spinning behind your window and look, the sky's a white glare in your window and

240

look, the sun's a white haze in the sky in your window and look, there's oil from your eyes and salt from your eyes floating like hairs on the sun in your window and look, there's blood on the walk hot under your feet before you slip on your shoes, before you turn to walk,

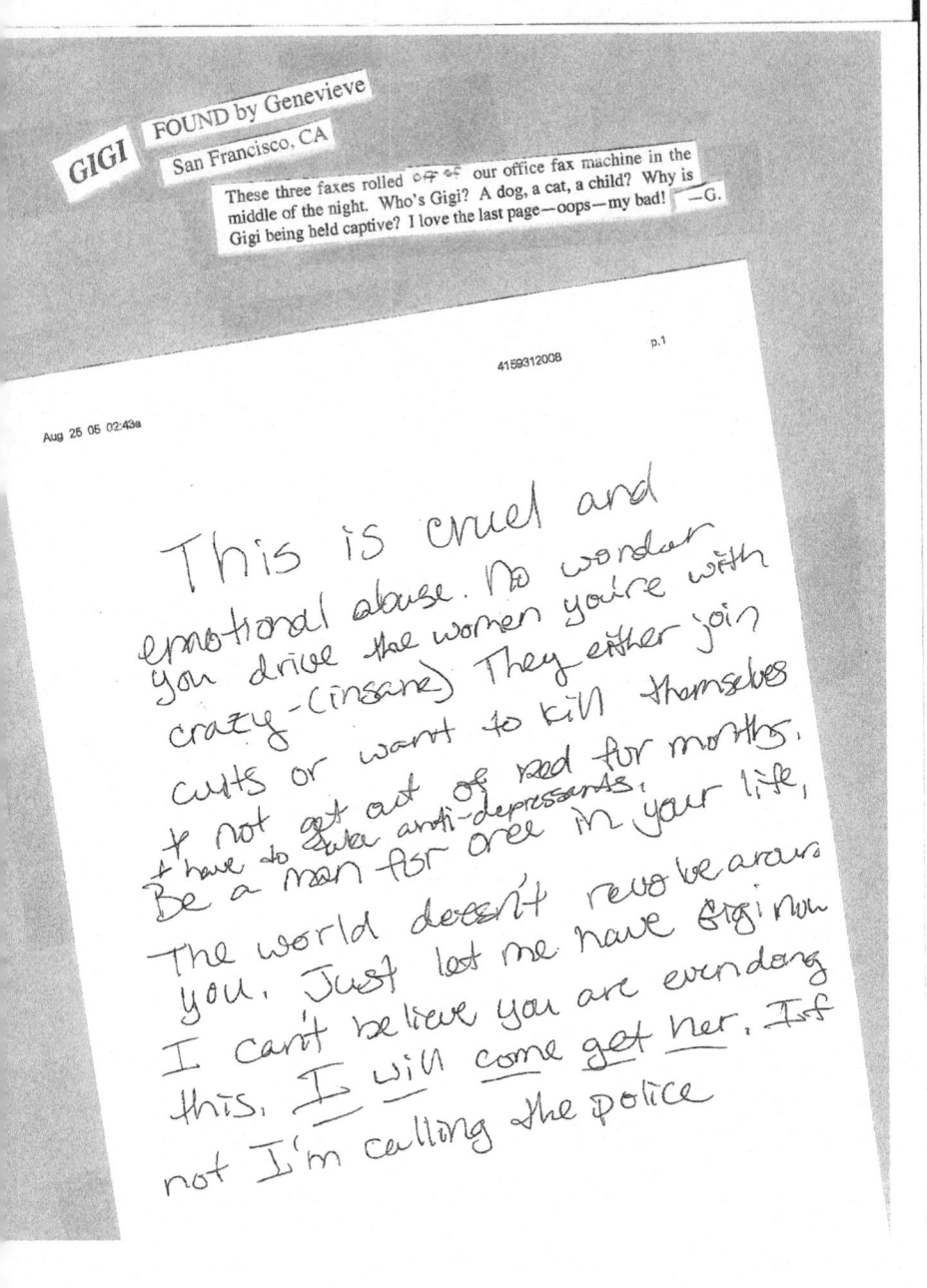

p.1

4159312008

Aug 26 06 02:43a

This is cruel and emotional abuse. No wonder you drive the women you're with crazy-(insane) They either join cults or want to kill themselves + not get out of bed for months, + have to take anti-depressants. Be a man for once in your life, The world doesn't revolve around you. Just let me have Gigi now I can't believe you are even doing this, I will come get her. If not I'm calling the police

FAX THIS! (OR, MY BAD)

COMPLIMENTS OF DAVY ROTHBART

AWAKE!

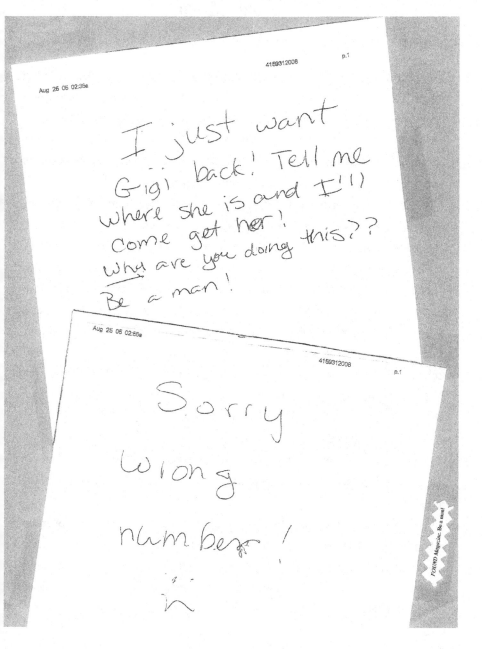

HOW INSOMNIA SAVED MY LIFE UNTIL THE NIGHT IT TRIED TO KILL ME

CLAIRE MOED

Before any of this ever happened, Sleep was a horrid sorrow—the day fading into some dusk, the trains going by and sounds of children being smacked giving way to sounds of adults being smacked. All I knew was there was heartbreak in that pink thing called the sky. Before I could think more about what made a soul hurt, someone would be shaking me awake and another day would begin, offering up its perils into my face and other punching spots on my body.

But like middle-age weight that creeps onto your thighs, insomnia crept into my life. It was the night of November 28, 1972. I was thirteen. Oh, now I understand the studies out of Minnesota that say something about teens needing to develop melba something or other and school needing to start later. But that's not what was happening. My insomnia was truly the stroke of a genius god who said, "You wanna know why this night is different from all other nights? The space to grow up as a person is officially and completely shot to hell, what with your junior high school's homicide rate (1—well, 1.5), your friends beating you up because they hate themselves, your mother unraveling into rage and your father's suicidal breakdown. But look, if you stop sleeping it will be the only time of the 24-hour cycle you don't get the shit kicked out of you by anyone. So is it a deal?"

And other than the couple of dozen times my nocturnal safety zone was interrupted by my father screaming his nightmares into a soft little pillow because his father came back in a coffin to yell at him, Night became the heaven I always dreamed about.

It was a win-win situation. With a pair of headphones and my small collection of cherished long-playing vinyl albums, I finally got the peace and quiet to imagine what I would have been like if only my real parents, those rich people from some big castle with ponies in New Jersey, had finally found me after that terrible mix-up at the hospital.

The fringe benefits of my new Night life were terrific. Besides beginning a life-long love affair with non-instant coffee, my daytime exhaustion became the legal and slightly less addictive tranquilizer I needed to not register how furious I was each time someone hit me with a word or a fist.

This perfect arrangement worked for several decades. I crashed through a lengthy adolescence of melodramatic self-sufficiency, and my twenties were filled with huge meals from the diner run by the Holocaust survivors on Tenth and Second, seventeen entry level jobs, ten years of undergraduate classes and an apartment that had twenty-six broken windows and—in the winter—no heat. As the years bled into one another, the space between my Night Girl and my Day Girl widened. It didn't matter to me that between the hours of 8 a.m. and 11 p.m., I was a lumbering mess of social gaffes hidden in huge men's shirts and beat up jeans that wouldn't become fashionable for another fifteen years. Night was when I became who I really was. Like Cinderella with a different curfew, Night Girl had a voice like Ethel Merman, a sprint like 007, Jean-Luc Ponty's musical abilities—and power. Oh yeah, lots and lots of power. Deep in New York's night of lonely neon and the shouts of lonelier drunks, I slipped on the old headphones and as the needle touched vinyl, God's finger touched Adam and I became.

Oh, I made brief stabs at sleeping—the anxiety about the world blowing up in a nuclear war interrupted my nights for a month in the mid-80s. I didn't want to be awake when they pushed the button so I listened to a Muzak All Night radio station hoping it would knock me out. It didn't. In fact, the only real sleep I ever remember getting in twenty years was one night at the home of the elderly Hasidic Jews in Boro Park. They had invited me for Seder not knowing I was raised a Reform Jew and had once, during a summer stint at a New Age commune, accepted Christ as my lord and savior (a decision well worth it at the time—the food was fantastic).

My observant hosts didn't want me traveling on a Shabbas-Yontif night and I had to sleep over in a basement room that had no windows. I suspect guilt for not enduring the faith my hosts had fought to save from Hitler was the reason I fell dead asleep for twelve hours. That or God knowing I couldn't start an argument about Zionism if I was unconscious. So. That was it. One night. One night out of 7,280 including leap years.

And then it all changed. On October 15, 1993 I fell in love. After a disastrous three-month attempt at domestic lesbian bliss, a smoking habit run amok, and a forty-two-page suicide tome in which my dead ex-boyfriend repeatedly said it was my fault he was dead, my Day World shattered the minute I saw the face of our new addition to the PR department. My dual existence came to a screeching halt.

And this love? He looked like an experimental Gene Kelly movie. He was an avant-garde tap-dance across the tundra of Mongolia. He was the softer colors of a Matisse. He was what I'd dreamt of all those seven-thousand-plus nights. However, here in Day World, he was dating one of Voltaire's descendents, and within seconds of our introduction, it was blatantly obvious to all present (the boss, three supervisors, and the other secretaries) he couldn't even stand my presence.

I knew this was a mistake. Not mine but his. Twenty years of seeing him in the dark had to account for something and it was up to me to make things right. If I showed him my true being, Night-Girl, then he would recognize me from the cosmic planes we lived on between I and 6 a.m.—and he would eagerly give up the legacy of French literature that people only read because it was going to be on the midterm.

But I was completely stymied as to how I would accomplish this. His arrival into the world of sunlight left me incapable of going to the ladies' room—which was right next to my cubicle—without detouring to the other side of the block-long office where he sat to ask if I could get him some coffee or herbal tea from the lunch room (a rotating selection each week!). His taciturn replies only left me yearning for more, and the tittering symphony from one hundred and thirty staff dedicated to your corporate health didn't stop me from damaging my bladder and ruining whatever hope there was that beneath the folds of my second-hand Brooks Brother shirts there beat the heart of his true love—a woman he must have dreamt about. Especially since he rarely had insomnia.

The human resources supervisor called me in to review my drop in productivity and my increase in socializing. Still I couldn't stop. Finally, I was given my third "warning" before suspension or being transferred to our offices in Queens (a place I hadn't been back to since that Mets game in 1986 where they won in the twelfth inning and then the strike happened).

But in need of food and shelter, I adhered to the written-in-stone rules—which I had to sign in front of the vice president and the company lawyer—that I would not, under any circumstance, converse with my love unless it was business, he initiated contact, or it was a medical emergency. (I insisted on that last part because medical and emergency were open to interpretation and I felt mine would hold up in court.) My compliance lasted several days until, hidden in a stall, I overheard the human resources supervisor telling the office manager that she couldn't wait until the love of my life got married and moved to the San Diego office. The wedding was in a week and a half. By two Mondays from now, he'd be gone, I'd be back to producing massive amounts of word processing, and she could cut back to only two bottles of Maalox a day.

My foot almost slipped into the toilet in shock. If this came to pass, my life would be over. I had to find a solution and I had to find it fast. Within an hour I was leaving work because my grandmother had died (again). I ran all the way to the East River and sat, frantically trying to come up with an algebraic solution. If this guy equaled my real life and my real life was me divided into the night but I only saw him in the day (fractions) and my day life was me minus my night life, then I had to add my night life to my day life. Which would eventually equal him equal me squared divided by nine. Well, six if you were in base eight.

The extra forty-five pounds I didn't have at Night and my firm belief that once I lost my day weight I'd look like Emma Peel were minor points. There were efficient pills out there and leather was only a second hand shop away. I'd be ready in no time. It was my personality I was concerned about. See, at Night I was Marlene Dietrich and Greta Garbo, only less verbose. In the Day I was a fucking canary. Chirp chirp chirp chirp until even I wanted to shoot myself. But I knew, knew that deep inside I had less to say and better words to say it. My true love and I had had devastatingly brilliant conversations for many years that if I had written them all down it would have brought back the film noir comedy. Could I shut myself up? And could I do it before he walked down the aisle?

That night as the records played, I stepped back and watched Night Girl. There she (or I) was—thin, dark, alluring, and funny. We were perfect. But where was the invisible force field that separated Day from Night? Where was the hidden portal?

And then at exactly 2:37 a.m., in the depths of a rendition of "Here's to the Ladies Who Lunch" by Stephen Sondheim, the mystery revealed itself. Night Girl was rested. She smiled like liquid chocolate pouring out of a vat. She moved like melting butter across a lukewarm skillet. She husked like she smoked two packs of unfiltered a day. So comfortable with herself, Night Girl could sit on an old wicker couch on some porch I had only read about in WASP literature and do nothing. The solution was obvious. In order to shut up I would have to sleep. At least one night.

I immediately cancelled all my weekend plans. Which wasn't hard. I had none.

But how could I make myself sleep? Pills were out because Jacqueline Susann never lied and all her heroines died from getting a good night's rest. The religious Jews in Boro Park were out because not only were they dead, they had found out from a neighbor who knew the cousin of a friend of my sister's accordion teacher that we used electricity seven days a week and played Wagner on our wooden recorders (but only once at the music school Christmas concert). So even if they weren't dead, it wouldn't have worked out.

That left hot baths and warm milk, both liquids that made me break out in hives. There was exercise. That made me PMS no matter what time of the month it was and the last thing I needed to be doing instead of sleeping was crying and eating. That left booze.

Well it worked for teething babies and drunks. Except for the fact I hadn't taken a drink in years.

It had all started with the fourth grade science project. It was Melissa's idea, really. After all she had the white mice. Jennifer could get wood, hammer, and nails from her brother Eric, who, unbeknownst to his parents, was building a space ship in his room. And I? I had Mother's secret stash. One bottle Manischevitz Grape Wine. The theory was that the white mice would make their way through a maze sober but would get lost if drunk. Pretty brilliant for a bunch of nine-year-old girls. Eric built the maze, but only because Jennifer blackmailed him with the threat that she'd tell mom and dad he was trying to run away from home via Mars.

That fateful fall day we carefully unpacked our tour de force in the school library. The mice were set carefully down in their obstacle course and I carefully brought forth the stolen wine. It was then that we realized we didn't have a way to feed our micies the booze. Melissa found a Dixie cup. We put one mouse up to the cup, but Stuart Little wasn't having it. The cup was too full, but we couldn't pour it back because we had already stuck the mouse's face in it. There was only one thing to do. I drank it. We tried to pour another cup down the mouse's throat, but that only soaked the mouse and Melissa's best shirt. I drank the rest of that too. Then we soaked a Twinkie in the cup. I drank that too and ate the Twinkie because the mouse didn't. By the time all our mothers and out-of-work fathers showed up to see our great progress in Madame Curie Land, I was legally intoxicated several times over.

My mother screamed at me in public that I was a drunk just like Bubby and how dare I steal my father's wine. I puked all over her B. Altman brown pumps. She never forgave me for that and I never drank again.

Until this night.

Why was this night different from all other nights? Was it because I was giddy like a bride before the piano started banging the wedding march, frantic like the Hebrews getting the hell out of Egypt, or desperate like a Monkee for the last train to Clarksville? All I knew was I had three nights to get sleep and five working days to stop my man from marrying the wrong woman, even if she did speak fluent Mandarin.

From what I gathered through my binoculars about the habits of night drinkers, 2 a.m. was a good time to pass out. For the first time in several decades, I turned off my record player and stepped out into the world I only knew about from looking through my window. With a pounding heart I headed to the all-night bulletproofed Plexiglas liquor store down on Fifth Street. I dashed, I skipped, I scampered. I danced by two drunk guys in the midst of an existential discussion that consisted of the single word "dude." I whirled around the six exhausted kitchen workers stumbling out of the overpriced delicatessen clutching leftovers for home and beers for the subway. I scuttled through the rats commuting from the construction site to the sewer. I hopped over the homeless guy who slept every night on the block he grew up on. And there I screeched to a halt. I stared at him huddled in the sleeping bag he got from the local born-again Christians. Maybe he had dreams too. Maybe he dreamt he'd wake up in his former home. Maybe I would wake up as Night Girl. Maybe, finally, we would both wake up as ourselves. Sleep as the cocoon from which the butterfly emerges.

There's a lot you can get with $23. I went for variety rather than quantity and the end result was an international medley of bottled sleep. Would I start with the Italian red, the Kentucky gold or the Russian clear? Would I sip or would I guzzle the German rum? Would I float into a bundled bliss or, like Bubby, crash to the floor oblivious and drooling? I broke every seal, grabbed all the coffee mugs I had gathered from all the stupid jobs I had lost, and started swallowing. If I got lucky I might even sleep a whole day AND night. Why, I'd not only be rested, I'd be thinner!

But the very thing that had harbored my dreams had also been the hidden room for my Anne Frank, the only place in the world where I saw myself loved and loving, the only one where I ever felt like a person, not a freak-show bull lurching through china shops (my one and only talent). My Insomnia turned around, ground me into the floor, and screamed in my face, "You fucking want to sleep—are you crazy—are you fucking crazy after all I have done for you?!!" And then with the rage of a woman who's been married to "that sonofabitch" for the best years of her life only to be told he's leaving her for his twenty-year-old secretary, my Insomnia picked me up and slammed me against the wall. And let me tell you, from that point on I was *wide* awake.

Wide awake and completely wasted. Walking a semi-straight line to the bathroom in the hopes of puking and passing out would have been a miracle out of Lourdes. Instead, my attempt at traveling from one end of my apartment to the other became a modern dance of smashing into different walls in different rooms. My homage to Fred-Astaire-with-a-coat-rack occurred when, in a feral leap to avoid yet another crash, I grabbed the twelve-foot bookcase and pulled it on top of me. It being 4:30 in the morning, two nights and one day after I had actually started drinking, my downstairs neighbor who hadn't spoken to me in seventeen years called me to tell me to stop making so much goddamn noise before slamming the phone down, aborting my desperate cry of help which sounded something like "arrrgguuhhaaaaa" but really meant "they shoot horses, don't they?"

Figuring the bathroom was a safe place to camp out for the duration of this new vicious awakeness, I managed to crawl out from under the many unread and very heavy books my father kept mailing me and drag the phone into my empty tub. It was the closest thing to a bed near the toilet just in case my Insomnia decided to surrender my body. Hope springs eternal.

Nothing but a massive alertness needed for microsurgery on severed limbs arrived, so I drunk-dialed every single person I knew, telling them how much I loved them. This included the pedophile camp counselor who got fired for visiting me at bedtime. I found him in Calgary where Canadian TV shows were much more polite to sex offenders, and I thanked him for his courage to risk his paycheck over my twelve-year-old company. He was touched but uninterested since I was now too old for him, fourteen being his cut-off date. The main goal—to sleep and to emerge anew like that Greek chick Persephone—didn't happen even with repeated doses from every bottle. And the more TIME ran out, the more I drank.

And then before I could count backwards from one hundred, it was Sunday night. My plan had failed. My one and only act, since that night in 1972, had utterly and unequivocally failed. I watched the moon—hazed by permanent pollution—rise. With each Night air molecule collapsing into yet another imaginary life I couldn't touch with my hands, my desperation blasted out of every orifice, clawing up my throat, pounding through my eyes, pouring out of my hair follicles: I will never be loved by the man of my dreams I will never be loved by the man of my dreams I will never be loved. What exploded through my body that night was but the soundtrack of all I had lived between the hours of I and 6 a.m. from the age of thirteen to the age of thirty-four crushed into a single long yowl of a life never accomplished in daylight. The wasted years and the lie I had become, a monster incapable of being who I really was, detonated and my head became a bomb slamming repeatedly against the bathroom wall and that's all I remember until I awoke three days later in a hospital bed.

The ICU nurse explained that neighbors above and below heard this scream, a keening they said that went on for hours. Since I had been such a quiet loner for so many years, they assumed that a) I was finally getting laid or b) somebody had died. Either way they didn't want to interfere. It was the huge thud sound abruptly interrupting the wailing that gave them pause, so they called the police, who broke down the illegal fire escape window gates and found me bleeding to death from a huge leak in my cracked skull.

My alcohol level was in frat party range, so medication and surgery were not options. I was put in the ICU under observation by a couple of interfaith chaplains ready to give last rites of any kind just in case I died, which was what they were all expecting.

They couldn't find any family information on me, but one of the cops discovered a pay stub under my bed and a social worker called my job looking for next-of-kin. That explained the generic bunch of carnations and get-well balloons from human resources next to my respirator. I guess if they thought I was going to live they would have sent real flowers.

There was a brace around my head to keep my brains from moving. The ICU was dark and quiet and the rhythmic machines that kept the heart attack guy stable and the organ donor alive long enough for harvest were soothing and after waking up and getting the facts I stopped remembering anything until the next time I opened my eyes and it was five days later. Without checking the date I knew the wedding was happening right then and there on some estate I should have grown up on but didn't. Instead I was in some dark room with more machinery than a NASA rocket. This was my life. This was my stupid life.

The organ donor was gone, off to be disseminated, I guess. The heart attack guy was still there, this time conscious and complaining to his wife who cried all over his face, telling him over and over again, "I love you, Morty. I fucking love you." I couldn't take my eyes off of them. As I watched true love for Morty, a kid arrived. Her family was nasty to the nurses, mean to the doctor, angry at her, but this kid just stared, like she was watching TV on some other planet. She stared like I had stared all those nights and I could tell she was beginning to weave her own great escape and it was going to last as long as it was going to last. It was then and there I knew my days and nights of being swaddled in fantasy and fear were over. I knew this because finally, twenty-one years, three months, and sixteen days later, I felt rested. I sent her a silent bon voyage. Good luck with your new world. Just don't stay too long or you might not get out alive.

Even with all the sick days I had accrued, I was fired for excessive absences. They sent a telegram to the ICU and the priest read it to me. Better than last rites he assured me. For several days I cried to whatever chaplain was on duty about how I had lost the love of my life because my love never met me after I had gotten a good night's sleep. The Episcopal reverend told me that if this was my true love he would find me again when the time was right and she knew because that's what happened to her and her wife when they met in seventh grade but then got married to the football captains of opposing teams in high school and didn't see each other until a class-reunion game years later. The Buddhist monk told me the Universe never says No. It says Yes. Yes, but not now. No, I have got something better. That's all the monk said. And the rabbi reminded me that in the concentration camps many often had to eat out of the same bowl they shat in and that sometimes life is like that. You eat and shit from the same bowl.

The social workers arranged lots of things and I didn't get evicted. I came home to a bathroom smeared with aged blood and old medical debris, and an apartment that had been raked over by the local crack addicts who'd slipped through the gates the minute the cops had left with the ambulance. The crackheads finished the booze and left behind the jewelry, the TV, my binoculars, and many empty vials.

However, as I stood before the entertainment center, I remembered what the monk had said about the Universe never making a mistake. Because the only things the crackheads *had* taken were my record player and every single one of my cherished long-playing vinyl albums. I stared at that sudden empty space for a long, long time. Finally, I cleaned up the blood, fixed the gate, and in that space where I'd once lived, I put the wooden bowl Bubby had grabbed the night she fled the Cossacks to a new world. Then I got into bed and slept.

HE SLEEPS ON
MATTHEW ROHER

Two hours of crying in his crib, then sleep.
Thin miserable snow again & dreams
of her beat against the windows in this
sharpened air: come home & be my blanket.
He sleeps on. Things around the apartment,
some of them, start to shimmer. Everyone
in their cars, driving at top speed outside.
He's still asleep, it's only been seven
minutes. I must keep myself awake or
be visited with horrors. Empty home.
My love hurtling toward me through vast subway
tunnels in one hour & twenty minutes.
Where am I now? I am a dream a black
obelisk dreams & forgets. I haven't
put much thought into it. I just feel good.

SATURDAY

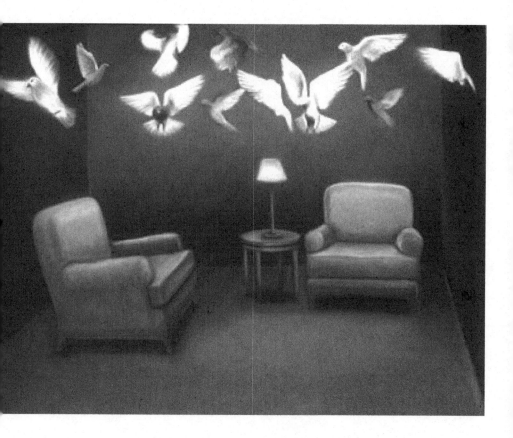

Sometimes a Fluttering Sound

A WOMAN STAYED AWAKE FOR THIRTEEN NIGHTS; AFTER THAT, SHE TOOK TO DRINK

ROSE GOWEN

On the first night she berated herself for not sleeping.

On the second night she exhorted with herself to get some rest.

On the third night she knitted a Fair Isle sweater.

On the fourth night she wrote sonnets to lost lovers.

On the fifth night she ripped her poems to pieces.

On the sixth night she drew silhouettes of her enemies.

On the seventh night she rearranged the furniture.

On the eighth night she tried threats and bribes.

On the ninth night she begged and pleaded.

On the tenth night she smashed her clocks and blacked out the windows.

On the eleventh night she cried.

On the twelfth night she sharpened her knives.

On the thirteenth night she plaited a rope from torn bed sheets.

THE PERIODIC TABLE
KAREN CONDON

The Periodic Table of Elements painted on my ceiling has kept me awake for the past seven nights. The guy who lived here before me painted it there. I don't know his name or what happened to him. He graduated. He moved on. He's in a better place now.

If I knew his name and where he was, I might get some closure. I don't know much about the Periodic Table of Elements, but it seems to me that it's about closure and nomenclature, two of the things closest to my heart. More things in life should be arranged in tables. There ought to be a neat separation between night and day, childhood and adulthood, one person and the next, just as there is between magnesium and sodium.

Radon. Beryllium. Titanium.

But even the elements don't stay in their boxes. There are reactions. Compounds are formed, bonds created and broken, heat released, energy transferred from substance to substance.

Only the two-letter symbols for the elements appear on the table. I photocopied and laminated a list of the names of all 104 elements from a chem textbook I still have from high school, and I'm going to memorize them. I like their sound. What they are and can do I have yet to learn, but I have nothing better to do until classes start in a week, such as sleep and eat like a normal human being.

"Don't you have anything better to do, man?" my roommate Mitch said to me this morning as I pored over the table. I'd known Mitch for exactly two days. Already I was sure I knew the only two aspects of his character that will ever matter to me: he gets right to the point, and he is unclean.

"I'm a chem major," I said without looking up. "Didn't I tell you?"

"No you're not," he said.

"How would you know?"

"You have the fuckin' *Norton's Anthology of English Literature* on the fuckin' coffee table, man."

"I'm switching."

"Come on. We've got a whole week. Shouldn't you be reading fuckin' *Beowulf* or fuckin' *Catcher in the Rye*?"

"I've already read *Beowulf* and *Catcher in the Rye*."

I glanced up furtively as he took a skillet out of the fridge, sniffed it, and slammed it on the stove.

"You're not a clean man, are you. Mitch?"

"Nope. I've got my priorities straight, that's why."

His current priorities appeared to be the proliferation, in this tiny apartment, of congealed animal fats and raw, gut-wrenching honesty.

Boron. Radon. Chlorine. Fluorine.

I decided I preferred the "ine" elements to the "on" ones. The "ilium" ones aren't bad, either. I let my head drop into my hands, just for a second, so I could think about this. When I opened my eyes again, Mitch had turned and was watching me.

"Hey, you want some eggs, man?" he said.

"No, thanks," I said.

"You gotta eat. You don't look so good."

"I ate already."

"Your cupboards are empty."

He turned back to the stove as the skillet began to smoke.

"That's because I ate it all," I answered.

"All I can say is, it's gonna be a long fuckin' semester," he said.

"Zirconium, zinc, yttrium, ytterbium, xenon," I recited as he cracked three eggs in the rancid skillet.

"Damn straight," he said.

He is a cheery enough guy, probably because he's so good-looking, in that suburban Aryan golden boy style. I am at once enchanted and repulsed by his beauty.

Mitch left for work still licking his greasy fingers. He closed the door quietly, as though not to wake me. I listened to his footsteps as he descended the fire escape to the sidewalk, where he kept his bike. When I was sure he was gone, I got up and stretched and opened one of my cupboards to look for something to eat. I had: 1) a package of Ramen noodles and 2) an unopened jar of peanut butter.

I leaned over the Periodic Table, muttering names of elements when they came into focus, abstractedly dipping chunks of noodles into the peanut butter and eating them. I tried to come up with mnemonics, but the words were other-worldly, and their abbreviations often unrelated to their names, so I opened the textbook and began to read.

As always, it started with history, men and their big ideas, same thing. Democritus opened the whole can of worms by naming his indivisible particles *atomos*. Plato and Aristotle gave him a hard time, but Democritus stuck to his guns. Joseph Proust and the *law of definite proportions*: compounds always have the same kind of elements stuck onto each other, in the same numbers. Dalton one-upped Proust with his *law of multiple proportions* and, my favorite, the *law of conservation of mass*: matter can't be created or destroyed. Something disappears, it just goes somewhere else, and you can either look for it or not look for it. "If you love something, set it free," and all that. Then J.J. Thompson and the cathode ray tube, and R.A. Millikan, who figured out the charge of an electron. Rontgen, Becquerel, Marie Curie, alpha, beta, gamma rays. Rutherford and his cohorts frolicked around the nucleus.

Their cover blown, protons, neutrons, and electrons appeared voluntarily like pilots shot down in enemy territory, and chemistry belonged to us.

I closed the book and momentarily found myself wandering around the apartment, peering into the other two empty rooms. I sat down on the sofa, turned the television on, and was instantly mesmerized by Judge Joe Brown, who was lambasting a skinny teenager who'd kicked in his neighbor's car door. *You better get your act together, son, because this ain't no way to conduct yourself as a young gentleman, do you hear me?* I nodded. During the commercial, waiting for Judge Joe Brown's verdict, I rested my head against the back of the sofa and examined the ceiling. It had been plastered over with a texturing tool in random, fascinating shapes. It was soothing to follow them with my eyes. I did that until my neck began to hurt, and looked up.

At some point, Judge Joe Brown had come to a close, and the soap operas had begun. I turned down the volume and watched the actors and actresses emote into each other's eyes, into telephone receivers, into thin air, and over gravestones, throwing practiced glances at the cue cards at opportune moments. With stricken expressions, ever so slowly, a blond couple drew closer to each other until their lips were touching, then turned their heads at complementary angles and kissed hungrily, as though in competition to consume one another's tongues. A middle-aged woman in a flowing turquoise pantsuit poured herself a drink from a crystal flask and paced her living room, talking and rolling her eyes. A gloomy, dark-haired man unwrapped a revolver from a monogrammed handkerchief and fondled it, smiling secretively: he had a plan.

"That ain't no way to conduct yourself, son," I said. I stood up and returned to the kitchen. It was now 2:30. Hours had passed silent as water. I opened *The Story of Chemistry* to where I'd left off.

I had just arrived at an explanation of how the Periodic Table is organized when Mitch returned from work. Looking at his glowing face—he was finishing a summer of lifeguarding—I felt suddenly exhausted.

"You're *still* on that, man?"

I ignored him.

"You appear to have gotten some more sun today, if that's possible," I observed.

"Yeah," he agreed, checking out his irradiated forearm. "Hey, six-fifty an hour, I better get something out of it."

He sat down across from me and slid the textbook over to his side of the table.

"You even talk like an English major," he said as he studied the page I'd been reading. "All fuckin' elegant, and shit."

He shut the book and stood up abruptly.

"You kill me, man," he said. "I need a shower."

I followed him to the bathroom and stood outside the door. I felt so lonely.

"When are Ben and Stan coming?" I called to him through the opening.

"Who?"

"You know, the new roommates."

"Their names aren't Ben and Stan, hey," he said. "They'll show up. We're all from the same town."

"You should've carpooled."

"I was working here all summer. They probably will carpool."

He didn't sound exasperated, though I wasn't making a whole lot of sense. He didn't seem to mind me standing there talking.

"Stan drives a Dodge Aspen," he continued. "Believe that? 1981."

"Yeah."

"What an asshole."

I nodded.

"Actually, just so you know, his name is Brian."

"And what about Ben?"

"Same thing, only with a *y* instead of an *i*."

AWAKE!

"How do you tell them apart?"

Mitch laughed, then, and I jumped a little, realizing I'd been nodding off against the doorjamb.

"Their names are the same, man, but they look different," he explained. "Get it?"

"They really should have different names," I slurred, turning away from the door by rolling my shoulder against the jamb. I slid along the wall to my room, where I tripped over the rug, went down on my knees, and crawled onto my futon mattress.

"Rutherfordium," I mumbled, settling my head on the pillow. "Einsteinium. Curium. Mendelevium."

I drifted on the surface of sleep. Each of these elements, I knew, was not only named after a different scientist, but is a unique combination of different kinds of molecules, each molecule with a different mass and size. They were never created and will never be destroyed. They are elemental. That last word dropped like an anchor behind my eyes.

I awoke completely contained by an unnamed night. I strained to see the ceiling, held my hand in front of my face, saw nothing. My eyes rolled playfully around, freed of their usual responsibilities, as I tried half-heartedly to recall where I was. A rhythmic thumping began in the adjacent room, accompanied by a soprano voice going, "ahh, ahh, ahh, ahh," and a tenor going, "aww, aww, ahah, aww, ahah, ahah." I recalled Mitch's flawless golden forearm as he reached for my book across the kitchen table and then I knew: I was at 241 Main Street, between the halfway house and the athletic supply store, and my pretty roommate, Mitch, was having sex with a girl whose name probably ended in "i."

I couldn't see it, but I knew the Periodic Table lurked on the ceiling above my bed, biding its time. I imagined it dropping on me like a net, the letters of the elements creeping all over me in a blind panic.

Moving my futon in the dark was not as difficult as one might think. My only other furniture is a dresser, which I keep in the closet, and some bookshelves. I got down on my knees and plowed the mattress across the floor until it met resistance. Then I crawled back on and slept.

When I opened my eyes to daylight, I found that I'd managed to push the futon up against the flimsy bookshelves, and that several paperbacks had fallen around my head. Morning sun from the window illuminated my feet. On the ceiling was a single crack, shaped like the coast of someplace. I traced it from end to end with my eyes. Now that, I thought, is something I can memorize no problem.

There was a clang in the kitchen as Mitch began his breakfast preparations. I listened for giggling or whispering or whatever sounds girls make in the morning, but she must have been asleep.

"Hey," Mitch said as I shuffled into the kitchen.

"Hey."

He rattled the skillet against the burner and swore.

"Long night?" I said.

He switched off the burner and sat down at the table. I sat down across from him.

"I brought home this girl."

I nodded, wide-eyed. Everything was so simple. It was morning. I was awake. My pretty roommate was talking about a girl. I had never realized how simple the morning could be. Mitch looked me over.

"What, did you sleep last night, or some such shit?"

"Yeah," I said. "I slept for hours. I moved my bed."

"Good idea."

"What's the girl's name?"

He sighed and ran his fingers through his bleached curly hair.

"I don't think she told me. I don't think *she* even knows. I met her at the pool. She looks like a fuckin' Coppertone ad. I didn't sleep all night."

"Coppertone," I repeated.

"Coppertone," he repeated, letting his head drop and desperately scratching his scalp with both hands. "I didn't sleep for even two seconds all night."

He flipped open the chemistry book, flipped it closed, and stood up abruptly. "But hey, I'm late, so you're gonna have to keep her company."

"Okay."

"Will you do that for me, man?"

"I'll make her breakfast."

I realized he'd probably never had insomnia before. He needed a crash course in sleepless living. I stood up and put an arm around his shoulders, guiding him to the door.

"Drink some coffee," I advised him. "Do everything more carefully than usual. Eat. Speak only when spoken to. Simplify, simplify, simplify."

AWAKE!

"Okay," he said, opening the door and stepping out onto the fire escape, his hair a ragged halo in the morning sun.

"I'll take care of Coppertone," I told him as he stepped slowly down the stairs. He stopped at the first landing and looked up at me with the insomniac's exaggerated earnestness.

"I know it," he said, blinking and shading his eyes. "I guess I better get my priorities straight."

He turned back and disappeared so quietly down the next flight of stairs it was as if I'd dreamed him.

I went back inside, sat down at the table, and opened *The Story of Chemistry*. The story of chemistry certainly doesn't have a linear plot, I thought, glancing affectionately over the Periodic Table. It had a definite though irregular shape, and an internal order that I'd been on the brink of learning the previous afternoon when Mitch had returned from work. I had to give the Periodic Table credit for trying to be symmetrical and predictable. It was like the face of an insomniac, placidly concealing internal ruptures, expansions and contractions, repulsions and attractions, desperate transfers of energy, broken bonds, on its pale surface expressing nothing beyond its own opaque nomenclature.

My stomach made an apologetic gurgling sound. I was hungry. I had no food left. I thought I must be hungrier than I'd ever been in my life. I got up and opened the fridge. Sitting on the bottom shelf was Mitch's skillet, with several broken pieces of bacon half-submerged in a hearty layer of congealed grease. I carried the skillet to the sink and scraped it out into the garbage disposal. I hit the switch, hoping that running the disposal would wake Coppertone.

Fifteen minutes later, the kitchen was a merry chaos of sound: sizzling bacon and eggs, the bottoms of my bare feet shuffling busily on the linoleum, the breathless bubbling of the coffee maker, my own voice as I sang what I could recall of The Who's "Pinball Wizard." I heaped food onto two plates and carried them to the table.

Wiping my hands on a dish towel, I listened for signs of life from Mitch's bedroom. But beyond the ticking of the stove element, my breathing, and the morning commuters' cars dragging themselves up the hill and into town, the apartment was still.

I hadn't realized how quiet it was here. You could think in this kind of quiet. I decided to eat my breakfast and let myself think instead of studying *The Story of Chemistry*. Different things occurred to me, lazily, one at a time: characters from books I'd read, scraps of poems, how my favorite professor paced restlessly around his office, smoking a cigarette without taking it out of his mouth, talking to me with his eyes closed.

I turned to Coppertone's plate when I'd cleared mine. I was still hungry. I decided to go check up on her, and if she was still asleep, to eat hers too.

I nudged the door to Mitch's room open with my toe. I'd never been in there. The bed was positioned in the center of the room, covered by an oversized white comforter that hung all the way to the floor. On the left side, on a single white pillow, lay a slender golden forearm, underside up, fingers curled delicately. I couldn't see the shape of her body under the thick comforter. Just the arm. Mitch had brought an arm home last night. He'd met an arm at the beach, and taken a liking to it, and now it was asleep on his pillow.

"That deaf dumb blind kid," I sang softly, "sure plays a mean pinball."

I backed out of the room.

I ate the arm's breakfast fast. It was getting hot in the apartment. I went out on the landing, stood for a moment in the glaring sun, and started down the stairs, thinking of swimming. I could go down to the town pool where Mitch worked, but I wouldn't. Instead, I got on my bike and headed for the pond.

The pond is deep, spring-fed, with trees gathered like patient spectators on the shore, some leaning out over the water. It's unguarded except by hand-painted SWIM AT YOUR OWN RISK signs. Take care of yourself here, in other words, because anything goes.

I swam out into the middle and floated on my back there, sculling with my hands, my breath loud in my ears, while swallows flew back and forth overhead as though erasing something.

I arrived home at sunset. As I pulled my bike behind the bushes and leaned it against the house, I heard voices next door at the halfway house, where two people sat across from each other at a picnic table, under a tree. One—the therapist, I imagined—sat back with his head tilted, his hand cradling one side of his face as if he had a toothache. The other person, whose back was to me, sat hunched over the table, rocking and leaning on his elbows. As I watched, the therapist stood up, carefully stepping backwards over the bench, went around the table, and waited patiently while his client also stood and awkwardly stepped over the bench himself. I turned and began to climb the stairs. As I reached the first landing, I heard laughter from above.

AWAKE!

"Aww, I'm okay, you're okay!" someone called. The therapist and his client turned and looked up at the third floor landing. I looked up there, and saw two more bronze towheads—Bryan and Brian—leaning on the railing and laughing. I put my head down and climbed the last flight.

When I reached the top, they'd gone into the kitchen, leaving the door open, and Mitch was angrily dragging his skillet over the stove.

"I'm *serious*, man," he said, whipping around, wielding the skillet. "One: this skillet is *cast iron*, morons, you don't just *wash* it, understand, idiots? Two: don't *fuck* with the people at the halfway house. Go outside and, fuckin', torture bugs instead."

I smiled, pleased with Mitch. He was feeling the truth-telling effects of insomnia.

Bryan and Brian glanced at each other and rolled their eyes.

"Psychopath," one of them mouthed to the other.

"Hey, I heard Dale Earnhardt Junior crashed his Corvette at NASCAR yesterday," said one of them. They went into the living room where they took over the sofa and the television, surfing the channels, searching for the explosive crash on the news.

"Earnhardt escaped, miraculously, with only minor burns," exclaimed the newscaster in a well-oiled voice. "How is that possible, Steve?"

I sat down at the table as Steve, his finger pressed over his ear, began his explanation.

"Hey, I'm the one who washed your skillet," I told Mitch. He was leaning over the sink, scrubbing the skillet, triceps bulging.

"Yeah, I figured. But they're idiots. I'll just scrape the rust off and oil it down."

"Is Coppertone still here?"

"Nope."

I listened to the scrubbing for a few minutes, until he let the skillet drop with a clang in the sink and turned around.

"You believe those shitheads, man?" he said to me. He had dark wings under his puffy eyes.

"Yeah," I agreed.

"They're here, what, fifteen minutes, and they're all in my face."

"I know."

"Shit."

I nodded.

"But look on the bright side," I said. "At least Dale Earnhardt Junior escaped with only minor burns."

He nodded. He laughed a short laugh and shuffled over to the table, dropping into the chair opposite me.

"Listen, let me cook you something to eat," I suggested. "Then you can help me finish memorizing the Periodic Table of Elements. That'll put you right to sleep."

"You're still on that, man?" he said, but he opened *The Story of Chemistry* to the Periodic Table on the inside cover and pulled out the laminated list of names, which I'd used as a bookmark.

"Don't you have anything better to do, man?" he murmured, his eyes running over the table as he saw it, really saw it, for the first time. I smiled nostalgically and turned to the skillet, realizing that things had come full circle, and that we would both sleep through the night.

INSIDE THE MIND OF AN INSOMNIAC
W. Bruce Cameron

I often lie awake at night worrying about the ill effects of getting too little sleep. Recent news has reinforced my concern; for example, scientists have discovered that when laboratory mice are deprived of sleep for an extended period of time, the little rodents have trouble performing certain tasks, like running mazes and operating heavy machinery. I have even read that not sleeping can cause you to gain weight, especially if you get out of bed in the middle of the night to eat a chocolate pie.

My problem is that my brain seems to come alive when I try to sleep, though it does a good job of being dormant whenever my editor calls to ask where my column is. Lying there, I wind up having an interior dialogue, like this:

ME: Okay, lights are out. Time to sleep.

BRAIN: Now would be a good time to worry about your credit card bills.

ME: No! There's nothing I can do about them right now.

BRAIN: I disagree. We can calculate how long it will take to pay them off, based on your current rate of debt reduction. I'm coming up with the winter of 2012.

ME: How is that supposed to help?

BRAIN: Our feet are itchy.

ME: What?

BRAIN: I've got a question. How do you explain the career of Ben Affleck?

ME: Just stop, okay? No more thoughts. Let's try counting sheep.

BRAIN: Do you think the People for the Ethical Treatment of Animals would be okay with that? I mean, sheep don't exist just for you to count them, you know. They have their own lives and worries, thank you very much. How'd you like it if someone made *you* into a sweater?

ME: Are you crazy? They're not even real sheep!

BRAIN: And that somehow makes it right? Hey, what does that roll of blankets at the foot of the bed look like to you?

ME: It looks like a roll of blankets.

BRAIN: Could be a snake.

ME: This is madness. How could a snake get in here?

BRAIN: A copperhead.

ME: There is no snake. Go to sleep.

BRAIN: Copperheads are poisonous, you know. *Shhh!* Listen!

ME: What is it?

BRAIN: I think I heard someone coming in the window carrying an axe.

ME: Oh for heaven's sake.

BRAIN: You should have asked Beverly Ballou to the Winter Dance.

ME: Wha— That was in seventh grade! Why are you thinking about that *now*?

BRAIN: I'm just saying. Sixty.

ME: You're just saying sixty?

BRAIN: I'm counting sheep, like you asked me to. I'm up to sixty. Are you sleepy yet?

ME: Yes! Let's go to sleep.

BRAIN: Beverly Ballou, you sure blew that opportunity. What a fool. We'll regret that forever. Have you noticed how much hair you've lost lately?

ME: I have not!

Brain: Okay, excuse me. The hair must be growing out of the shower drain, then. What are you worried about, anyway? Bald men are considered "very sexy" by focus groups comprised primarily of bald men.

ME: I am not going bald.

BRAIN: Maybe you should get up and check in the mirror. Hey, what are the symptoms of the Ebola virus? I think we've got it.

ME: We're not getting out of bed, we're going to lie right here and go to sleep.

BRAIN: Oh yeah right. Did you remember to turn off all the burners on the stove?

ME: Yes, I did.

BRAIN: Are you sure? I think I smell smoke. You cheated.

ME: I . . . huh?

BRAIN: High school algebra class. You looked over and saw Todd Smith's answer for question number four. How can you live with yourself?

ME: I didn't mean to!

AWAKE!

BRAIN: It's not too late to set the record straight. I'll bet you we could track down our teacher. What was her name? Waters? Rivers? Something wet. Mrs. Drip Faucet? Mrs. Dribble Drink? Can you seriously not smell something burning? I can practically hear the flames.

ME: Fine!

When I get up to check the burners, I usually raid the refrigerator. (As long as I'm not sleeping, I figure I might as well get a chocolate pie out of it).

ME AND THE GOLEM
GARY LUCAS

For many years, I've had an intense, intimate relationship with the Golem.

What I mean is, for over a dozen years now, I have been assiduously working with the 1920 Paul Wegener/Carl Boese silent film *Der Golem—How He Came Into the World*, having composed a score to accompany it live on electric and acoustic guitars, played in real time through many secret electronic effects (no samplers or sequencers here). The sound is symphonic, the science-fiction flavored music sumptuous and mystical.

I've played with this film in over fifteen countries around the world since debuting it in 1989 with my original keyboardist/collaborator Walter Horn at the BAM Next Wave Festival in NYC. Since 1993, I have been working with the Golem in a solo format. Tel Aviv, London, Berlin, Budapest, New York, San Francisco—all have felt the power and majesty of the Golem again, as I reanimate this film—a big hit worldwide upon release—with my own spectral music. I never grow tired of it. Night after night, it's like peering into a telescope at a microcosm of 16th century Prague, the Jews stooped and shuffling their way through Hans Poelzig's gnarled and misshapen ghetto mise-en-scène like some fantastically garbed Mummer's parade, strolling the streets and moving into the synagogue for evening prayers. I love witnessing the dramatic arc of the story unfold time and time again, the tale of the actual historic Rabbi Jehudah Loew and his Kabbalistic magical prowess, and how he created the Golem, a man molded from shapeless clay, to become a servant of the Jewish people, to protect them from annihilation—the ultimate revenge for love of his daughter Miriam as the Prague ghetto is consumed by flames, caused by a Golem run amok. I delight in the foppish antics of the lustful Junker Knight Florian, the sly machinations of the servile sorcerer's apprentice Famulus, and Wegener's all-too-human portrayal of the hulking juggernaut, the Big Fella himself—Go Go Golem! Each night I play my heart out into this black and white phantasmagoria, changing the music round every time I perform it, improvising new shrieks, whispers and sighs on my guitar, curdling new electronic frissons in my electronic cauldron, hurtling my Jewish heavy-metal soul across the yawning chasm of eighty-some-odd years to try and put some spring back into the Old Boy's feet of clay. I have played my music to this film literally hundreds of times, and I never get tired of it, I keep seeing new things within it, and it keeps haunting me, keeps drawing me back.

My absolute favorite city to perform the Golem in, bar none, is Prague, of course. (My roots are literally Bohemian, and my family name was once Lichtenstein, "stone of light"—Lucas is close to that, deriving from the Latin root for luminous ... true to my name, I like to throw light in dark corners.) I've played it there many, many times, beginning with a performance in the Reduta Jazz Club (where Bill Clinton previously held forth with his saxophone) in 1993. And also, most memorably, in the cavernous crumbling old Yiddish theater known as the Roxy, near the Mala Strana section of Prague's Old Town Square.

Let me tell you about one such memorable performance: It took place in the unusually hot (for Northern Europe), stifling summer of 1995. I had been summoned to Prague by a fellow musical eccentric named Richard Mader, who goes by the name of Faust, himself an underground rock legend in Czech progressive music circles, and the owner of his own label Faust Records. Faust had proposed to record a collaborative album with me and his band Urfaust on the theme of "The Ghosts of Prague," after seeing me play solo in Prague earlier that year. He had been full of praise for what he enthusiastically described in a letter to me as my "ghastly" guitar stylings. To that end, he had secured me several nights at the Roxy performing *The Golem* to pay for my trip to Prague, and had secured a good print of the film from the Goethe House archive for me to play to.

This gig was fraught from the beginning.

Faust, a six-foot gentle giant of a fellow with a perpetually cheery outlook (a good counterbalance to my own mercurial weltanschauung), arrived at noon at my Dresden hotel the day of the first scheduled Golem show, having driven the normally three-hour trip from Prague to East Germany in his battered Skoda to come and personally fetch me there. He excitedly showed me the Czech newspapers full of previews for my Golem engagement, and mimeoed flyers announcing the same, chattering on in his charmingly fractured English about the crazy album we were going to make together and the stellar gig I would perform solo that evening. ("It's gonna be a sold-out house, of that I am sure! Because we work on PROMOTION! We work on PUBLICITY!" "We" meaning Faust Records, his pride and joy—which consisted solely of him and his long-suffering assistant and mistress, Marta. They had come to visit me in NYC that spring and had spun grandiose plans of Czech music-world domination.) And after stuffing the boot of his old car to capacity with my guitars and my dreaded, cumbersome Monster Case full of electronic effects (which he christened "The Flying Mary"—the scourge of many a European tour manager), we were off on a hot, sweaty, endless journey to Prague which took a maddeningly slow seven hours to complete, due to massive road repairs on an East German highway infrastructure which had been built before the War and hadn't been upgraded since. Also due to Faust's propensity for circuitous shortcuts, which unfailingly put us back on the highway, after much time spent stopping to consult outdated maps, in front of the shortcut exit we had just taken. "BOOL SHEET!" he would invariably spout, commenting on his own handiwork. "BOOOL SHEEET!"

We arrived, finally, literally by the seat of our pants, at dusk in Prague—the Magic City glistening in the fading light like a fairytale, the most beautiful city in the world, the spires of the St. Vitus Cathedral pricking the sky, rising over the green Petrin hills, the lights of the Charles Bridge winking at us as we raced past the imposing stone edifice of the National Museum, past the faded elegance of the old Railway Station, roaring up onto the elevated highway above the bustling thoroughfare of Wenceslas Square, epicenter of the Velvet Revolution, Faust frantically gunning our red bomber filled with my magician's wands and bag o' tricks, past the late Saturday crowds of tourists and shoppers, into the seedy heart of the old Jewish Quarter—where we finally came to rest in front of the run-down, fabled Roxy Theater.

We had less than an hour before showtime.

In great haste I set up my gear in front of the old screen, a remnant from the venue's Yiddish Theater days, checked the projection, tested the amps, all the while cursing Faust and his unerring tardiness, then stumbled solo out of the Stygian depths of the empty cinema into Prague's magic night. I picked my way down the twisting twilight streets to make an homage and pay my respects to someone very special to me through a short visit to the celebrated Jewish cemetery, nestled nearby the Roxy in the old Jewish Quarter at the foot of the Alte Neu Synagogue, which, legend has it, is the final resting place of . . . the Golem.

They sell postcards of the Golem all over Prague. A definite Favorite Son, no doubt about it. My brother the Orthodox Rabbinical student swears that he resides there still, in that Old New synagogue, in a locked attic room, rendered immobile until needed again, and that, with a special inscription on his brow writ by an Unseen Hand ("Emeth." as in the Golem film I love and play to, the Hebrew word for

Truth), or the rendering of certain obscure Kabbalistic rituals (reciting the Hebrew alphabet backwards, perhaps, as suggested in several scholarly tomes I've consulted), or through some recondite ritual unknown to current scholars, the Golem will rise, must rise, again. (It's said that during the Nazi occupation of Prague, when German SS officers entered the holy tabernacle of that Synagogue one night to desecrate the ancient Torah scrolls and pilfer the wealth of the holy relics displayed there, the Golem was awakened from his 400-year-old slumber. In the morning light that shone through the stained glass windows of the Alte Neu Synagogue the following day, the bodies of the Nazi soldiers were discovered, literally ripped asunder by some malevolent Goliath with superhuman strength. My brother, the Harvard graduate, swears by this tale.)

As the sky grew darker, and the midsummer night came on strong, I threaded my way over the winding stone pathway of the old Jewish Cemetery, through the thicket of ancient graves, pushing past some straggling Dutch tourists struggling with their guidebooks. Ah, here at last was what I'd been searching for.

Jutting up from the earth, they were—from the vaulted caverns below, sepulchers mouldering in this haunted burial ground, running twelve or so levels deep, caskets stacked up one atop the other because the original Jewish population were denied a decent plot of land to bury their dead in, so they had to make do, as always, as best they could—jutting skyward, all weathered black granite with nearly indecipherable inscriptions, looking like the broken, rotting teeth of some fallen giant, were the tombstones. I made for the biggest, blackest one.

Festooned with yellowing paper messages, like the tattered prayers stuffed between the cracks in the Wailing Wall, Rabbi Jehudah Loew's gravestone had become a repository for the hopes and dreams of all the wandering Jews who had made their way to his final resting place in Prague—"Please, Rabbi Loew, heal us as a nation"; "Please, Rabbi Loew, let little Rachel walk as normal children do"—and I too had a message for him.

Hastily I scribbled my prayer on the back of a printed flyer announcing my evening performance—"Please, Rabbi Loew, let the Golem rise again"—and placed it reverently at the foot of the weathered stone marker. The wind that sprang up then almost blew it away. But I caught it just in time, and tucked it firmly between a crevice in the headstone base and the rich, loamy earth of the old graveyard.

You never know.

My show that night was one of the wildest, most maniacal Golem performances I ever delivered—this was, after all, Prague—and I played as a man possessed, a madman, full of the scorn and fury of the ancient Hebrew patriarchs. I literally became as one with them, as in *Der Golem's* famous film-within-a-film sequence, wherein Rabbi Loew summons up a vision of the Jews in exile trekking across the desert, their grizzled Moses-like leader striding angrily off the screen into the theater/ Hapsburg Court to wreak vengeance on the terrified throng of skeptical, laughing spectators, my three guitars summoning a host of wraiths and malignant phantoms from the Kabbalah and Jewish lore to rise anew—Azrael, Astaroth, Lilith, Metatron, Habal Garmin aka "Breath of Bones"—all filling the empty vessel of the old theater with their shrieks and imprecations, spirits of the earth and air, writhing once again, to dance triumphant in the flickering shadows.

And then it was over. The giant Star of David symbol came up superimposed on the film's final shot of the old Prague Ghetto's shuttered gate, as my last harmonic guitar flourish, a strange dischord which is my signature "Golem motif," rang out in the packed, airless theater. "Don't you wish you had a Golem?" I shouted into the mic—my stock line at the film's finish. I got no answer this night, not the usual tumultuous, rapturous applause. The lights were raised, dimly. The audience, what I could make out of them, looked numbed, shell-shocked. And that's how I felt, too.

In a trance, in the kind of hypnotic daze my own playing sometimes puts me, I began to slowly pack up my guitars, operating on auto-pilot. Usually at this point I take questions about the film, the music, and the Golem legend from the audience—but not this night. I vaguely became aware of a crowd of people gathering at the lip of the stage where I had just performed, and where I customarily sell CDs of my music after the show.

"Hey man, your music was louder than the movie!" some wisecracking American student smirked. "Do you know what I mean?" he went on, covering his ears.

"Cool," I replied, "a little pain is good for you." Fuck off, buddy. (I am nothing if not . . . loud. I want to make you sweat with my music. I want to give you an orgasm with my guitar.)

Most of the crowd that had gathered, however (basically a motley assortment of Bohemian art intellectuals and various foreign tourists), were genuine fans, extremely enthusiastic in their response to both the film and my music, and I sold them many copies that night of my *Skeleton at the Feast* album, which contains my Golem score. There were a few cuties there as well, including one pouting zaftig

blonde in a purple leather getup that seemed molded to her skin, with holes stra-
tegically placed over and under her hefty Czech breasts, but I was too drained to
do much about it.

There was one face in that crowd though that really got my attention.

A skinny, prematurely wizened kid with sunken, haunted eyes, a severe,
near-skinhead buzzcut, and a crimson slash of a mouth, kind of like Klaus Kinski's.
He looked about eighteen going on eighty. He fixed me with his beady stare, and
beckoned me over to him at stage left where he had positioned himself in the
front of the crowd of onlookers.

"Meester Geddy Loookis," he spoke directly to me in that strange, deliberate
mittel-European Czech intonation that always reminds me of Peter Lorre. "I come
from a family whose mutter and fadder were both kilt inda kemps . . ."

Instantly my heart went out to this strange apparition. A landsman, I thought.

"End I just wanna say dat in your museek for dis film, I hear MURDER!! I hear
VIOLENCE!!"

He went straight for the jugular then, eyes popping at me accusingly,
self-righteously.

"End we Jews, you know . . . we . . . we just don't NEED this!! Not no more! Not
after de kemps! We haf to heal, you know? We haf to heal the world! NOT wid this!"
he spat at me.

Trumped by his survivor's status, fatigued from playing a wild, heartfelt show to
a strangely lackluster crowd, stifled by the airless cinema, and momentarily at a loss
for words, not at all my usual glib self, I mustered a subdued reply:

"My European relatives were killed too during the war, in a pogrom in Poland . . .
I play what I feel. And I feel angry about it still. And this film," I gestured back towards
the looming screen, "mirrors my feelings exactly."

"We don' need it here, unnerstand me?! Not your anger! NOT your hatred!"

He shook his head, turned his back on me, and walked off slowly in disgust.

Profoundly depressed by this excoriation of my art, my life, my raison d'être,
from someone with whom I otherwise sensed an underlying deep kinship, I packed
up the rest of my gear as hurriedly as possible in the now nearly-empty cinema
and went looking, unsuccessfully, for Faust, in order to collect my fee for the night's
performance.

The typical option of going back to the hotel to sleep was absolutely out of
the question. I was wired, livid, and adrenalized by both my performance and my

post-gig encounter with the midnight denizens of the Roxy. Facing the prospect of a lonely room and an empty bed was not an option that appealed at all to me at the moment.

Often I would treat my post-gig insomnia with a dose of Ambien and wake up after a half-restful unsatisfactory sleep a few hours later, bleary-eyed and ready to make the schlep to the next town.

But my nerves were too jangled to submit to a chemical solution.

Not this night.

I told one of the theater managers to keep an eye on my guitars and the Flying Mary for me, as I needed at that moment to escape the oppressive tomb of the Roxy as quickly as possible, to be alone with my shattered thoughts. I slunk, deflated and dejected and fighting successive waves of dizziness, out the rear stage door and into the oppressive Prague night.

I found myself in a darkened alleyway of slippery cobblestones, choking on the stench and the overflowing clotted refuse of open trashcans. I could barely see where I was going, there was very little illumination, no streetlamps shone back here, and I stumbled forward bumping into a slime-coated wall, rounding what seemed to be a corner in this warren of alleys, groping my way towards a glowing ember hovering in the distance, inching towards what I thought was the end of the alley.

The ember was the tip of a lit cigarette. Its owner stood not at the entrance to the street, but in front of a blackened wall, a cul-de-sac.

A dead-end street.

"Excuse me," I blurted, "I don't speak Czech. Can you please show me how to get to the street?"

The smoker, a shapeless black hulk in the dark, took a drag on his butt.

"Do you know how to get to the main street?" I said again slowly, plaintively. Like I said, I was a little bit dizzy.

"Street is dat way . . . come, I show you," the phantom said in a harsh, low voice. He tossed his cigarette, deliberately, like a spark shooting out of a crackling fire—then suddenly a convulsive movement and my arm was gripped by a relentless, tightening claw.

"You Jew musician from New York . . . I know you play here . . . tonight . . . I see newspaper . . . FUCK YOU JEWS! GO BACK AMERICA!!" the lout rasped at me as I recoiled from his fetid drunken breath. I tried to tear away from his manacle-like grasp, to wrench my arm away; managed to take a swing at him, connecting only

AWAKE!

with air. There was a short, brutish struggle and then I was seized by his sharp pin-
cer-like fingers and hurled down onto the slimy cobblestones, a sharp pain lancing
through my right forearm as I put my hands out rigid in front of me to protect my
head. I heard the click as of a knife blade opening, then felt the whistle of cold metal
tearing through my loose suitjacket shoulder, seeking my flesh. The knife rent right
through the fabric, narrowly missing my shoulderblade, ripping through the flimsy
summer jacket before striking the stone pavement.

"Goodbye, Jew ..."

I closed my eyes. I prayed to Yaweh. I prayed to Rabbi Loew for my deliverance.

I heard him laugh and whisper maniacally, "I am Breath of Bones!!!", heard him
sing out exultantly, again, felt his shrouded form pounce on my back, pinning me
down, hot breath on my neck, stabbing through the noisome air, clutching the knife.
Up for the downstroke—

Suddenly a sound of heavy boots.

A feral, guttural growl.

And I felt my phantom assailant literally torn from my back.

And with a whooping, echoing scream dissolve into the night sky.

I opened my eyes to discover Faust standing over me with a flashlight.

"Gary, Gary my friend, I been lookin' all over the theater for you ... my God
what are you doin' kissing the ground like dat? Did you slip or trip or somethin'? Bool
Sheet! Bool SHEET! Come on, I got your money, let's get the guitars and the Mary
and get the hell outta here ..."

I whispered one last prayer, mentally, to Rabbi Loew, then let Faust help me up
from the pavement where I lay. Gingerly cradling my right arm, I let the big Czech
drag me, limping, down the street, his boots beating a mighty tattoo in time with
my heart.

You never know ...

INSOMNIA
MARK MIRSKY

"Insomnia, the gift of the Divine (should the Unknown as Conscious Design exist), to the scribe."

This was the single sentence he did not erase from blocks of text on the screen of his machine, ephemera flying off into its vacuum, for the past three hours. He had hesitated at "scribe," wondering whether to choose "writer," flipping back through a thick tome on the nature of patches or additions through manuscript redactions of *Genesis*, checking sources on the role of the scribe in the Biblical book's transmission. Weary, before his screen, he licked up the last golden drops from the rim of a glass of old malt Scotch. "What dreams may come?"

He prayed aloud, "Come to me!" Awaiting intoxication, the slow drip of honey which allow him to go on through an endless sweetness of effortless paragraphs, he stared at his first effort, smeared obscene on the glass, mocking him with its sly reference to the World Beyond.

What do you want—to be swept up in the body? He tried to recall a pornographic DVD—the stamina of two men a young woman pumped like a busy bee. The image of the girl desperate to "satisfy" (he suspected it was all "pretend,") depressed rather than uplifted him. Now he felt no desire, or inspiration, only impure. Twice he had cycled through the academic text on scribal additions, searching for a moment to enter a Biblical place. Its scholar quoted lines from *The Book of Joshua* and a parenthesis about the boundary of the tribe of Benjamin, running to the slope of Lutz, *"And the border went over from there to Lutz, toward the slope of Lutz, which is the same as Beth El (today)."* The text's clarification implied the presence of a copier acting as an editor who contributed to the topographical reference, mentioning that a contemporary name for ancient Lutz was Beth El.

The scholarly note about Lutz suggested that the scribe's hand could be seen elsewhere, the man thought. A similar highway sign appears before the Biblical patriarch Abraham as he goes to seek out a place to bury his wife, Sarah, when she dies

AWAKE!

in Kiryat Arbah on the road, or resting, temporarily. "Kiryat Arbah, the place which is the same as Hebron in the Land of Canaan," states the text of *Genesis* as transmitted for several millenniums. Why was the scribe permitted into the story?

*

Had he prepared himself to receive, to *transmit* an idea? Or did he betray his calling, reaching the last drop of malt? What itch had carried him into the stretch of the morning past midnight? An hour ago, before the computer ticked past 12 a.m., he had felt drowsy, ready to sleep. Now he was passing the point when he could stagger onto his futon and collapse.

*

His prayer was a paean to exhaustion, "O seek me in this moment," he cajoled, desperation tinged with melancholy, self disgust, when a buzz, a bizarre incandescence jolted each and every limb. His body crackled, awake. Was he outside of time? I have passed—not "through the looking glass," he thought—but a clock face, its numbers reversed. An image turned gracefully on the glass, motioning to him out of a stream of silver blue flashes.

She (the beams had coalesced) laughed. The sound could have been his fingers over the keys, pattering as if they were agents of another's intention. A soft, tickling, brush touched his ear, though it was impossible to distinguish yet, exactly what *her* form was, dancing before him, or whether it was clothed or not.

"Who are you?" he asked, as if the image was not a trick of light and imagination. If he read the pixels correctly, she put a finger to her lips and indicated that he type his questions, even while wavering on the screen she seemed to read or understand the words that his mouth spoke to the screen.

"Why?" he picked out key by key the word, a thrill that carried back through his hands on the soiled plastic indentations to flesh recumbent in the chair, a charge that turned his seat's axis, swiveling below him."

"Don't you want to touch me?" Her lips moved on the barrier of glass, and an echo of them tingled in his ear.

"Yes," he said aloud, his voice mocking him as it bounced back from the screen. Her mischievous features were now distinct. He could read in the sideways tilt of her chin that he had violated the instructions she had offered. His fingers found the keys and typed out the three letters just spoken.

As if in response the figure on the screen showed herself to the professor in full length. Was she reclining on a couch? He did not recognize the flowing yet diaphanous robes but they did not entirely hide her prominent breasts or the rippling line of her long legs. Though it passed in a flash, he thought she turned her body so that he could imagine the twin halves of her bottom like the split of a pear that his mother once cut, two perfect opposites of a sphere, and lifted to tease him from a boiling pot of sugar syrup when he was four, five.

"Do you want a taste?"

This time he typed the three in a daze.

*

"Where are you from?"

Several times before he had woken in bed, unable to sleep in the interruption of a dream—between the time of a dream and the moments of a restless night. The idea of slumber sailed through the too watchful hours, oblivion an elusive cloud even as he reclined. If he were very careful not to fully awake, the fantastic events in which just moments before he had been gripped, would knit themselves back into scenes and move to a form of resolution. The dream would continue, even though its fragile links had been broken and certainly altered by his rising close to consciousness (this could not be helped) but could in altered form, resume when he sunk back into its drama.

Now, between waking and intoxication, nodding before the screen, his lips moved without sound in a dumb show of articulation, his fingers gliding over the keyboard.

It did not surprise him when the young woman answered his question in Hebrew. Happily he recalled the Biblical phrase, "*Kiryat Arbah, which is the same as Hebron.*"

"Which one?"

She laughed softly so that her breath clouded the glass before him.

"Which?" He repeated his question.

"Always," she answered, coming close so that he felt the air she exhaled now, tickling his nose with specks of sage and mint crumbled into dust, "the former."

Her breasts stiffened against the glass, their nipples pressed almost painfully in a smudge of pink to where his fingers waited to trace them as he tentatively reached to explore an uncertain surface.

"Do you wish?" she asked.

"Yes," he whispered, "let me . . ."

Her voice however came from behind him. "Find me!"

*

Had he slept momentarily? *"Kiryat Arbah, which is the same as Hebron."*

He recalled her voice again and the verse of geography she spoke. It was intoned in an accent so peculiar, harsh, as if blowing in the wind, or the wind blowing through the syllables, that he wondered for a moment if the speaker were not Arab, bringing a different set of accents and breath to words that had cognates in many Semitic languages.

The girl from Kiryat Arbah could be a Palestinian. Was she—like those who had eyed him narrowly on his trips through the Arab towns of the Holy Land, recognizing his Jewish mannerisms under the costume of a tourist—hostile? Could she be a religious Israeli, the light of Biblical prophecies revolving in her sharp gaze, one of those fanatical settlers willing to die for the sake of a damp crypt?

Understanding his dilemma, it seemed, the young woman, again pressed her breasts against the glass. He heard her laugh in back of him, just as he watched her nipples pop out of the robe, rub back and forth, as if tempting his fingers to seize them through the glass.

"How old do you think I am?"

Her lips just by his ear, tickled it and he felt fingers lightly touch the sparse white hair of his head.

"I am not a child of the Hebrews or the Palestinians. My tribes lived in the 'City of Four' before your father Abraham wandered west from Haron." She giggled. "What magnificent hair you have."

*

"You flatter me," I responded.

"No, you are so handsome, tonight."

"I'm old . . ."

Her voice broke into my apology. "How old do you think I am?"

"Nineteen, twenty,"

I felt the pleasure come leaping up in me like the breaking of a *djinn* from a jar in long stoppered. Wind, lightning and thunder, a quickness flashed in every limb as if I too could spring as I once did on my toes, whirling in a storm, bounding, imitating a stag. For a moment I felt myself brush her nakedness, the small firm buttocks and the swell of her belly above the thighs. I too was bare before her.

Her breath was full of perfume, though, slow and sticky. I went dizzy when I heard or thought I heard her say, "I am older than you."

"How much?"

Her voice was low, and her small breasts, cool to the touch but rigid as their enflamed tips as I held them in the hollow of my palms, "Millenniums."

Her flesh felt like an adolescent's.

Was she, however, older? Would these delicate bubbles that promised to root in my body, burst out in ruddy red, orange, yellow—springs of childbirth, shooting color through their tips, shrivel instead against a skeletal frame at the first stray ray of dawn? Dawn, was my link to the planet and its clock. Was she a nightmare?

"Time," her voice tipped into my ear, "has another logic in your dreams, the past world flees back to the present."

"Nothing is lost?"

"Nothing you can imagine," she replied.

"Have I imagined you?"

"You could never imagine this." She lay back on the narrow bed beside my desk.

Instead of a flowing robe that costumed her form in the flat dimensions of the screen, she wore a pair of shorts. An empty bottle of wine and the remains of a flask of cognac sat on the computer desk a few feet away.

"This is so constricting," she muttered undoing the belt of her shorts, then putting her thumbs under the band of her underwear.

I divested myself of my own clothes but she had fallen asleep, and barely stirred when I embraced her.

*

He was at a loss to explain the situation.

"Wake up," he whispered.

"Why?" she asked, without opening her eyes.

"Otherwise, I will think that I am dreaming."

"It is I, who am dreaming," she answered.

"Why?"

"You wanted me."

He was awake, and yet the apparition was as real as his wife across town, the bedroom in the five-room flat, their children, snug in bed.

He ran his hand across her naked back, admiring the strong rib cage, the narrow waist, the firm proportions of a small tapering seat, its perfect halves.

What do you want from me? he wished to ask, but seemed as if it would dispel the mystery between himself and her.

"Take me," she whispered.

Had he heard the words, he wondered, but when he bent to her the body under him was without passion, half asleep, and for a moment when she seemed to rouse herself playful it was as if he, not she, were the toy.

"Take me ..."

"Where?" he asked, lying next to her now, but depleted of the will to enjoy whatever desire might lurk in the long body next to him, naked in his sheets.

"Anywhere but where I am."

"Where is that?"

"You were searching for images. Imagine the world of Kiryat Arbah."

*

It was a lacuna in the Biblical text, a place with a history before Abraham, a measureless past, whose Hittites mingled with the aboriginal inhabitants and tribes drifted in from the wide open spaces to the south and east.

"I can't."

"Imagine a cave," her voice invoked its space, musty, "smelling of cooking fire smoke, animal hide, damp wool, urine, jars of honey, dry grass and spearmint, chamomile ..." He was drawn into her amusement. She rubbed against him until her body unloosed a bouquet of lilies, gardenias, and carnations. They filled the room together with the raw odors she had mentioned.

"Why do you think Abraham brought her body here?"

Here? He meant to ask where that was, but light filled the room, pouring through the screen. He was awake but blind in its brilliant wash.

"How old do you think the Pharaoh thought Abraham's wife was?"

She touched him, tenderly, taking hold of his private part, in long, tentative fingers. The gesture did not inspire lust but tenderness, a daughter's caress against his cheek, a mother's, stroking his hair.

"How could Pharaoh guess?"

"Who brought you here?" he asked.

For a moment she was the nubile matriarch, Sarah, in the king of Egypt's chamber. "I already answered," she whispered, but her hand had withdrawn.

"Your wish is holy."

The prelude to a deep sleep fell like a heavy blanket over his arms and legs drew him into her folds. As if about to drift into the sweetness of union, oblivion, and prophecy *Tardemeh*," he thought, recalling the Hebrew syllables for that mantle of slumber. Waiting, lying back, slowly he realized, although weary, that he could not close his eyes.

*

She was sleeping. Regarding the length of her, it was an image of all he could desire but still distant, so that he found it impossible, considering this, to be next to her. Drowsily he lifted him himself back to his feet. A taste that suggested dates bursting in the sun filled his mouth. He recognized the artifacts of his room, the narrow bed, a chair, but inhaled the scents of another place as he drew a sheet over her body. It is a rite, he thought, I must, according to the rules, withdraw.

What was Sarah's time like in the bed of the king of Egypt, or again in the boudoir of Avi-melech, monarch in the midst of Canaan? Both men returned her intact, half afraid of what they had been close to.

What did the dusty town hold beside a burial cave, a hole into which three of the patriarchs descended to lie there beside a wife?

"I am older than Sarah," she said. He was by himself, apart, recumbent upon a couch, when he heard her voice again. His bones were heavy, leaden, but still he was not asleep.

"How old are you?" she teased. "In my world, Sarah is still a girl."

When would he know that this was a dream, that he was not awake?

"Do you think that Abraham ever passed a night without sleep? Did he brush the form of a forbidden union? Did he enjoy her, golden, as the kings had?"

*

Her fingers touched the flask of liquor. She was sitting up. He stood over her, dressed again.

"How did I lose my underwear?" she asked, as if she were moving through another time, far away.

Was Pharaoh frightened, as terror of the Unknown moved through him? Later the beguiling hostess of Jericho, Rachab, would tell the Hebrew spies who came to her that all the kings to the north and west had lost their juice, gone soft, helpless. A nameless dread moved through their towns, fortresses. Her nakedness, which previously had provoked their organs to a frenzy of appetite, now reduced the commanders to damp tears, shrunken endearments.

"I love images of horror," she said, gathering her clothes, undergarments scattered under feather pillows, a woolen blanket. He went down on his knees to help her search behind the bed.

AWAKE!

"Recite a poem," she ordered, sitting on the lip of his narrow resting place, pouring a drink for herself, its last intoxicating beads.

*

Like a coward, afraid of what he has seen, the man turns his back, shuts himself off from images in his chamber, and creeps toward the bleaker light that begins to radiate through the eastern window of the rectangular space in which he sat all night, then stood, and then again, reclined.

The scribe hears the voice in the Pharaoh's ear, "It will cost you dear to return to sleep."

The light promises sleep, whereas the night that lies behind him is the wall of dreams, shadowy shapes, the gaudy paintings of caves and pyramids on which the creatures of the old stories flit: lie in wait, promising a final insomnia. There one's eyes will close perhaps against the distractions of this world.

"Take me . . . ." Does she mean it, or is it his own hallucination, the drop of liquor in his brain? Why does he press himself against the window, afraid? What has moved against him in the dark?

ARCHITORTURE

SHANNON WHEELER

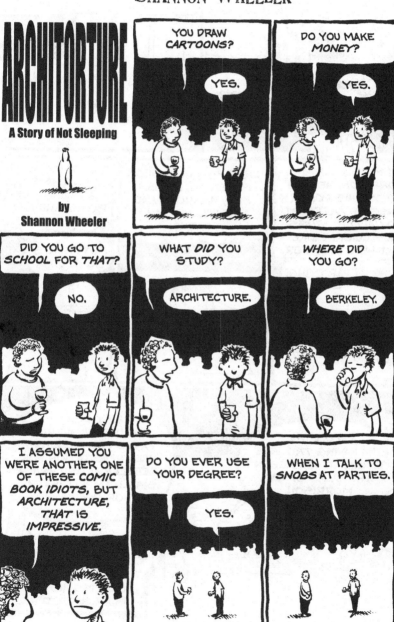

IT'S TRUE. *BEFORE* I STARTED CARTOONING I STUDIED *ARCHITECTURE* AT UC BERKELEY. THE PROJECTS WERE LONG, INVOLVED, AND USUALLY REQUIRED A *SLEEPLESS* NIGHT OR TWO.

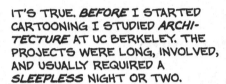

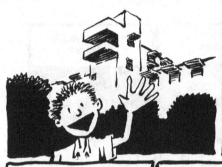

I WANT YOU TO *DESIGN A PARK* BASED ON THE *IDEAS* OF AN *ARTIST* YOU ADMIRE.

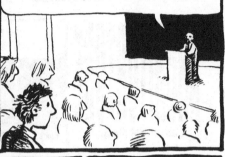

I'M USING *JIM MORRISON*, HE WAS A *GREAT*; HIS *POETRY*, SENSE OF *FREEDOM*, *SEXUALITY*, *DRUGS*, REBELLION. I LIKE WHAT HE STOOD FOR.

PARTYING.

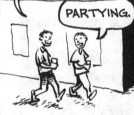

CRAP. HOW DO I SHOW *FREEDOM, DRUGS, SEX, ANARCHY* AND *REBELLION* IN A PARK?

THE *OBVIOUS* THING IS TO HAVE WILD PLANTS, WANDERING PATHS, AND A PLACE FOR POETRY...

BUT THAT'S SO *STUPID.*

EXCUSE ME, I'M HAVING *TROUBLE* TRYING TO REPRESENT THE *IDEAS* OF JIM MORRISON.

WHY DON'T YOU USE WANDERING PATHS FOR *FREEDOM*, WILD VEGETATION FOR *REBELLION*, AND HAVE A SMALL AMPHITHEATRE FOR *POETRY*?

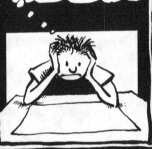

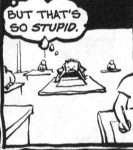

MY TEACHER, GETTING HIS *PH.D* IN ARCHITECTURE.

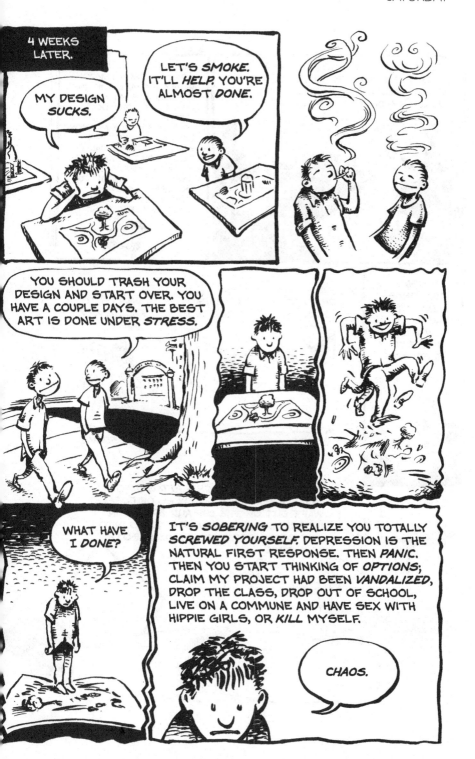

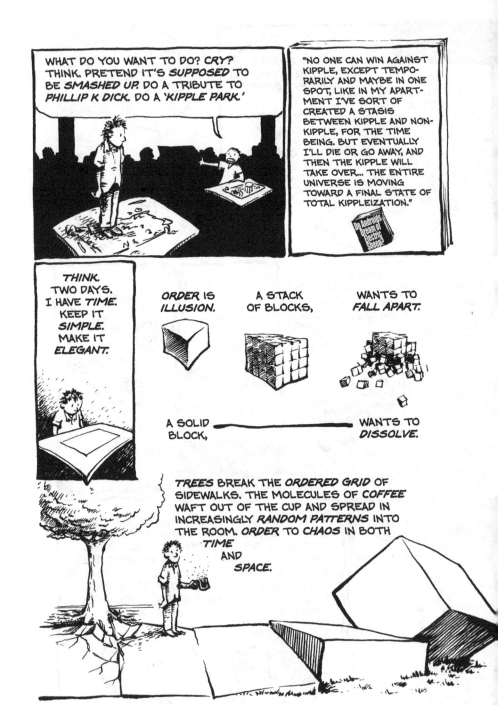

WHAT DO YOU WANT TO DO? CRY? THINK. PRETEND IT'S *SUPPOSED* TO BE *SMASHED UP*. DO A TRIBUTE TO *PHILLIP K DICK*. DO A *'KIPPLE PARK.'*

"NO ONE CAN WIN AGAINST KIPPLE, EXCEPT TEMPORARILY AND MAYBE IN ONE SPOT, LIKE IN MY APARTMENT I'VE SORT OF CREATED A STASIS BETWEEN KIPPLE AND NON-KIPPLE, FOR THE TIME BEING. BUT EVENTUALLY I'LL DIE OR GO AWAY, AND THEN THE KIPPLE WILL TAKE OVER... THE ENTIRE UNIVERSE IS MOVING TOWARD A FINAL STATE OF TOTAL KIPPLEIZATION."

THINK. TWO DAYS. I HAVE TIME. KEEP IT *SIMPLE.* MAKE IT *ELEGANT.*

ORDER IS ILLUSION.

A STACK OF BLOCKS,

WANTS TO *FALL APART.*

A SOLID BLOCK, ———————— WANTS TO *DISSOLVE.*

TREES BREAK THE *ORDERED GRID* OF SIDEWALKS. THE MOLECULES OF *COFFEE* WAFT OUT OF THE CUP AND SPREAD IN INCREASINGLY *RANDOM PATTERNS* INTO THE ROOM. *ORDER* TO *CHAOS* IN BOTH *TIME* AND *SPACE.*

THE DESIGN IDEA CAME QUICKLY. A GRID OF CUBES WOULD MAKE A SMALL PLAZA. *ORDER.* AS YOU WALK DOWNHILL THE CUBES WOULD SHIFT, TURN, AND RISE UP OUT OF THE GROUND RANDOMLY. *CHAOS.* *ORDER* TO *CHAOS* REPRESENTED *SPACIALLY.*

IN THE PLAZA, AT THE CENTER OF THE ORDERED CUBES, A *TREE* WOULD GROW. OVER TIME ITS ROOTS WOULD BREAK THE CEMENT. THIS WOULD REPRESENT *CHAOS* OVER TIME.

ENTROPY PARK, A TRIBUTE TO PHILLIP K DICK.

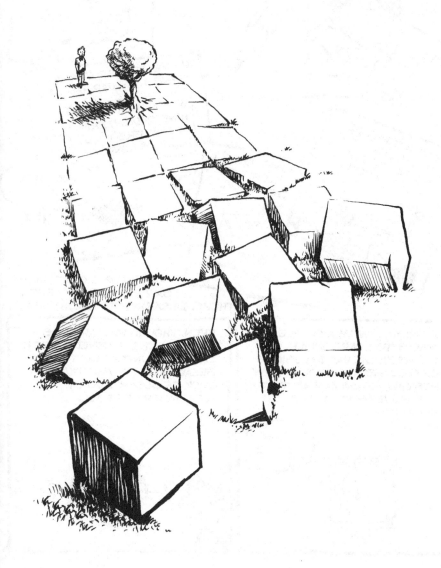

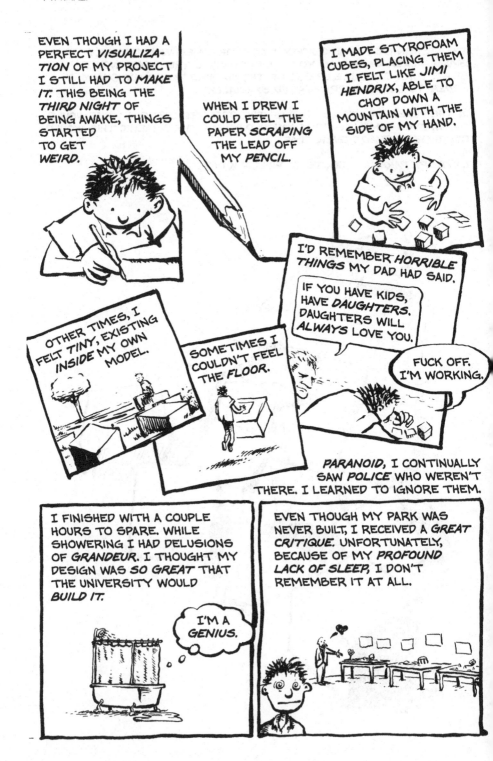

EPILOGUE

WE WENT TO A FRIEND'S HOUSE TO *RELAX*. I WAS *RANTING*.

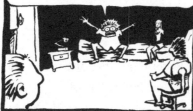

I *LOVE* IT! I DID A 6-*WEEK* PROJECT IN 3-*NIGHTS* AND I GOT A *BETTER GRADE* THAT *ALL OF YOU!*

IT'S BECUAUSE YOU *SLEEP* TOO MUCH. SLEEP MAKES YOU *WEAK*.

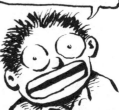

I'VE BEEN UP FOR *THREE DAYS* AND I FEEL *GREAT!*

SLEEP *DENIES* US OUR *SUBCONCIOUS*. THAT'S WHERE OUR *POWER* IS. IT'S AN *OCEAN* OF CREATIVITY. LET THOSE WAVES COME UP AND *SURF THAT SHIT.* WE'RE *ALL GENIUSES!*

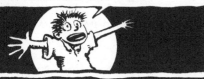

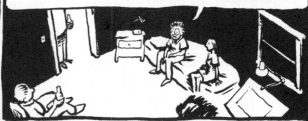

I WANT TO START MY NEXT PROJECT *RIGHT NOW!* I'LL *KICK ASS* ON THAT ONE TOO!

I DON'T NEED SLEE...

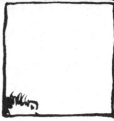

I WAS SO *RIDICULOUS* THAT MY FRIENDS THOUGHT I WAS *JOKING*. I SLEPT FOR *18 HOURS*.

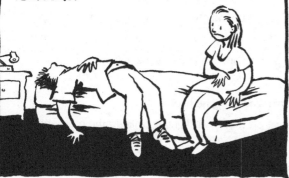

IT WAS THE *BEST* ARCHITECTURE PROJECT I'VE EVER DONE.

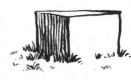

END.

I-80 NEBRASKA, M.490–M.205
John Sayles

This is that Alabama Rebel, this is that Alabama Rebel, do I have a copy?"

"Ahh, 10-4 on that, Alabama Rebel."

"This is that Alabama Rebel westbound on 80, ah, what's your handle, buddy, and where you comin from?"

"This is that, ah, Toby Trucker, eastbound for that big O town, round about the 445 marker."

"I copy you clear, Toby Trucker. How's about that Smokey Bear situation up by that Lincoln town?"

"Ah, you'll have to hold her back a little through there, Alabama Rebel, ah, place is crawling with Smokies like usual. Saw three of em's lights up on the overpass just after the airport there."

"And how bout that Lincoln weigh station, they got those scales open?"

"Ah, negative on that, Alabama Rebel, I went by the lights was off, probably still in business back to that North Platte town."

"They don't get you coming they get you going. How bout that you-know-who, any sign of him tonight? That Ryder P. Moses?"

"Negative on that, thank God. Guy gives me the creeps."

"Did you, ah, ever actually hear him, Toby Trucker?"

"A definite 10-4 on that one, Alabama Rebel, and I'll never forget it. Coming down from that Scottsbluff town three nights ago I copied him. First he says he's northbound, then he says he's southbound, then he's right on my tail singing 'The Wabash Cannonball.' Man blew by me outside of that Oshkosh town on 26, must of been going a hundred plus. Little two-lane blacktop and he thinks he's Parnelli Jones at the Firecracker 500."

"You see him? You see what kind of rig he had?"

"A definite shit-no negative on that. I was fighting to keep the road. The man ain't human."

"Ah, maybe not, Toby Trucker, maybe not. Never copied him myself, but I talked with a dozen guys who have in the last couple weeks."

"Ahh, maybe you'll catch him tonight."

"Long as he don't catch me."

"Got a point there, Alabama Rebel. Ahhhh, I seem to be losing you here—"

"10-4. Coming up to that Lincoln town, buddy. I thank you kindly for the information and ah, I hope you stay out of trouble in that big 0 town and maybe we'll modulate again some night. This is that Alabama Rebel, over and out."

"This is Toby Trucker, eastbound, night now."

Westbound on 80 is a light-stream, ruby-strung big rigs rolling straight into the heart of Nebraska. Up close they are a river in breakaway flood, bouncing and pitching and yawning, while a mile distant they are slow-oozing lava. To their left is the eastbound stream, up ahead the static glare of Lincoln. Lights. The world in black and white and red, broken only by an occasional blue flasher strobing the ranger hat of a state policeman. Smokey the Bear's campfire. Westbound 80 is an insomniac world of lights passing lights to the music of the Civilian Band.

"This that Arkansas Traveler, this that Arkansas Traveler, do you copy?"

"How bout that Scorpio Ascending, how bout that Scorpio Ascending, you out there, buddy?"

"This is Chromedome at that 425 marker, who's that circus wagon up ahead? Who's that old boy in the Mrs. Smith's pie-pusher?"

They own the highway at night, the big rigs, slipstreaming in caravans, hopscotching to take turns making the draft, strutting the thousands of dollars they've paid in road taxes on their back ends. The men feel at home out here, they leave their cross-eyed headlights eating whiteline, forget their oily-aired, kidney jamming cabs to talk out in the black air, to live on the Band.

"This is Roadrunner, westbound at 420, any you eastbound people fill me in on the Smokies up ahead?"

"Ahh, copy you, Roadrunner, she's been clean all the way from that Grand Island town, so motormotor."

(A moving van accelerates.)

"How bout that Roadrunner, this is Overload up to 424, that you behind me?"

(The van's headlights blink up and down.)

"Well come on up, buddy, let's put the hammer down on this thing."

The voices are nasal and tinny, broken by squawks, something human squeezed through wire. A decade of televised astronauts gives them their style and self-importance.

AWAKE!

"Ahh, breaker, Overload, we got us a code blue here. There's a four-wheeler coming up fast behind me, might be a Bear wants to give us some green stamps."

"Breaker break, Roadrunner. Good to have you at the back door. We'll hold her back a while, let you check out that four-wheeler."

(The big rigs slow and the passenger car pulls alongside of them.)

"Ahh, negative on that Bear, Overload, it's just a civilian. Fella hasn't heard about that five-five limit."

"10-4 and motormotor."

(Up front now, the car is nearly whooshed off the road when the big rigs blow past. It wavers a moment, then accelerates to try and take them, but can only make it alongside before they speed up. The car falls back, then tries again.)

"Ah, look like we got us a problem, Roadrunner. This uh, Vega—whatever it is, some piece of Detroit shit, wants to play games."

"Looks like it, Overload."

"Don't know what a four-wheeler is doing on the Innerstate this time of night anyhow. Shun't be allowed out with us working people. You want to give me a hand on this, Roadrunner?"

"10-4. I'll be the trapper, you be the sweeper. What we got ahead?"

"There's an exit up to the 402 marker. This fucker gets off the ride at Beaver Crossing."

(The trucks slow and the car passes them, honking, cutting sharp to the inside lane. They let it cruise for a moment, then the lead rig pulls alongside of it and the second closes up behind inches from the car's rear fender. The car tries to run but they stay with it, boxing it, then pushing it faster and faster till the sign appears ahead on the right and the lead truck bulls to the inside, forcing the car to squeal off into the exit ramp.)

"Mission accomplished there, Roadrunner."

"Roger."

They have their own rules, the big rigs, their own road and radio etiquette that is tougher in its way than the Smokies' law. You join the club, you learn the rules, and woe to the man who breaks them.

"All you westbound! All you westbound! Keep your ears peeled up ahead for that you-know-who! He's on the loose again tonight. Ryder P. Moses!"

There is a crowding of channels, a buzzing on the airwaves. Ryder P. Moses!

"Who?"

"Ryder P. Moses! Where you been, trucker?"

"Who is he?"

"Ryder—!"

"—crazy—"

"—weird—"

"—P.—!"

"—dangerous—"

"—probly a cop—"

"—Moses!"

"He's out there tonight!"

"I copied him going eastbound."

"I copied him westbound."

"I copied him standing still on an overpass."

Ryder P. Moses!

On 80 tonight. Out there somewhere. Which set of lights, which channel, is he listening? Does he know we know?

What do we know?

Only that he's been copied on and around 80 every night for a couple weeks now and that he's a terminal case of the heebiejeebs, he's an overdose of strange. He's been getting worse and worse, wilder and wilder, breaking every trucker commandment and getting away with it. Ryder P. Moses, he says, no handle, no Gutslinger or Green Monster or Oklahoma Crude, just Ryder P. Moses. No games with the Smokies, no hide-and-seek, just an open challenge. This is Ryder P. Moses eastbound at 260, going ninety per, he says. Catch me if you can. But the Smokies can't, and it bugs the piss out of them, so they're thick as flies along Nebraska 80, hunting for the crazy son, nailing poor innocent everyday truckers poking at seventy-five, Ryder P. Moses. Memorizes your license, your make, and your handle, then describes you from miles away, when you can't see another light on the entire plain, and tells you he's right behind you, watch out, here he comes right up your ass, watch out watch out! Modulating from what must be an illegal amount of wattage, coming on sometimes with "Ici Radio Canada" and gibbering phony frog over the CB, warning of ten-truck pile-ups and collapsed overpasses that never appear, leading truckers to put the hammer down right into a Smokey with a picture machine till nobody knows who to believe over the Band anymore. Till conversations start with

AWAKE!

"I am not now nor have I ever been Ryder P. Moses." A truck driver's gremlin that everyone has either heard or heard about, but no one has ever seen.

"Who is this Ryder P. Moses? Int that name familiar?"

"Wun't he that crazy independent got hisself shot up during the Troubles?"

"Wun't he a leg-breaker for the Teamsters?"

"Din't he use to be with P.I.E.?"

"—Allied?"

"—Continental Freightways?"

"—drive a 2500-gallon oil tanker?"

"—run liquor during Prohibition?"

"—run nylons during the War?"

"—run turkeys during Christmas?"

"In't that the guy? Sure it is."

"Short fella."

"Tall guy."

"Scar on his forehead, walks with a limp, left-hand index finger is missing."

"Sure; right, wears a leather jacket."

"—and a down vest."

"—and a lumber jacket and a Hawaiian shirt and a crucifix round his neck."

"Sure, that's the fella, medium height, always dressed in black. Ryder P. Moses."

"Din't he die a couple years back?"

"Sheeit, they ain't no such person an never was."

"Ryder P. who?"

"Moses. This is Ryder P. Moses."

"What? Who said that?!"

"I did. Good evening, gentlemen."

Fingers fumble for volume knobs and squelch controls, conversations are dropped and attention turned. The voice is deep and emphatic.

"I'm Ryder P. Moses and I can outhaul, outhonk, outclutch any leadfoot this side of truckers' heaven. I'm half Mack, half Peterbilt, and half Sherman don't tread-on-me tank. I drink fifty gallons of propane for breakfast and fart pure poison. I got steel mesh teeth, chrome-plated nose, and three feet of stick on the floor. I'm the Paul mother-lovin Bunyan of the Interstate system and I don't care who knows it. I'm Ryder P. Moses and all you people are driving on *my* goddamn road. Don't you spit, don't you litter, don't you pee on the pavement. Just mind your p's and q's and we won't have any trouble."

Trucks pull alongside each other, the drivers peering across suspiciously, then both wave hands over head to deny guilt. They change channels and check each other out—handle, company, destination. They gang up on other loners and demand identification, challenge each other with trivia as if the intruder were a Martian or a Nazi spy. What's the capital of Tennessee, Stomper? How far from Laramie to Cheyenne town, Casper Kid? Who won the '38 World Series, Truckin Poppa?

Small convoys form, grow larger, posses ranging eastbound and westbound on I-80. Only the CB can prove that the enemy is not among them, not the neighboring pair of taillights, the row of red up top like Orion's belt. He scares them for a moment, this Ryder P. Moses, scares them out of the air and back into their jarring hotboxes, back to work. But he thrills them a little, too.

"You still there, fellas? Good. It's question and answer period. Answer me this: do you know where your wife or loved one is right now? I mean really know for sure? You been gone a long time fellas, and you know how they are. Weak before Temptation. That's why we love em, that's how we get next to em in the first place, in't it, fellas? There's just no telling what they're up to, is there? How bout that Alabama Rebel, you know where that little girl of yours is right now? What she's gettin herself into? This minute? And you there, Overload, how come the old lady's always so tired when you pull in late at night? What's she done to be so fagged out? She ain't been haulin freight all day like you have. Or has she? I tell you fellas, take a tip from old Ryder P., you can't ever be certain of a thing in this world. You out here ridin the Interstate, somebody's likely back home riding that little girl. I mean just think about it, think about the way she looks, the faces she makes, the way she starts to smell, the things she says. The noises she makes. Now picture them shoes under the bed, ain't they a little too big? Since when did you wear size twelves? Buddy, I hate to break it to you but maybe she's right now giving it, giving those faces and that smell and those noises, giving it all to some other guy.

"Some size twelve.

"You know how they are, those women, you see them in the truckstops pouring coffee. All those Billie Raes and Bobbie Sues, those Debbies and Annettes, those ass-twitching little things you marry and try to keep in a house. You know how they are. They're not built for one man, fellas, it's a fact of nature. I just want you to think

AWAKE!

about that for a while, chew on it, remember the last time you saw your woman and figure how long it'll be before you see her again. Think on it, fellas."

And, over the cursing and threats of truckers flooding his channel he begins to sing:

> In the phone booth—at the truck stop
> All alone,
> I listen to the constant ringing—of your phone.
> I'd try the bars and hangouts where
> You might be found,
> But I don't dare,
> You might be there,
> You're slippin round.

They curse and threaten but none of them turn him off. And some do think on it. Think as they have so many times before, distrusting, with or without evidence, hundred-mile stretches of loneliness and paranoia. How can they know for sure their woman is any different from what they believe all women they meet to be—willing, hot, eager for action? Game in season. What does she do, all that riding time?

> I imagine—as I'm hauling
> Back this load.
> You waiting for me—at the finish
> Of the road.
> But as I wait for your hello
> There's not a sound.
> I start to weep,
> You're not asleep,
> You're slippin round.

The truckers overcrowd the channel in their rush to copy him, producing only a squarking complaint, something like a chorus of "Old MacDonald" sung from fifty fathoms deep. Finally the voice of Sweetpea comes through the jam and the others defer to her, as they always do. They have almost all seen her at one time or another, at some table in the Truckers Only section of this or that pit stop, and know she's a regular old gal, handsome looking in a country sort of way and able to field a joke and toss it back. Not so brassy as Colorado Hooker, not so butch as Flatbed Mama, you'd let that Sweetpea carry your load any old day.

"How bout that Ryder P. Moses, how bout that Ryder P. Moses, you out there, sugar? You like to modulate with a me a little bit?"

The truckers listen, envying the crazy son for this bit of female attention.

"Ryder P.? This is that Sweetpea moving along about that 390 mark, do you copy me?"

"Ah, yes, the Grande Dame of the Open Road! How's everything with Your Highness tonight?"

"Oh, passable, Mr. Moses, passable. But you don't sound none too good yourself, if you don't mind my saying. I mean we're just worried sick about you. You sound a little—overstrained?"

"Au contraire, Madam, au contraire."

She's got him, she has. You catch more flies with honey than with vinegar.

"Now tell me, honey, when's the last time you had yourself any sleep?"

"Sleep? Sleep she says! Who sleeps?"

"Why just evrybody, Mr. Moses. It's a natural fact."

"That, Madam, is where you are mistaken. Sleep is obsolete, a thing of the bygone ages. It's been synthesized, chemically duplicated and sold at your corner apothecary. You can load up on it before a long trip—"

"Now I just don't know what you're talkin bout."

"Insensibility, Madam, stupor. The gift of Morpheus."

"Fun is fun, Ryder P. Moses, but you just not making sense. We are not amused. And we all getting a little bit tired of all your prankin around. And we—"

"Tired, did you say? Depressed? Overweight? Got that rundown feeling? Miles to go before you sleep? Friends and neighbors I got just the thing for you, a miracle of modem pharmacology! Vim and vigor, zip and zest, bright eyes and bushy tails—all these can be yours, neighbor, relief is just a swallow away! A couple of Co-Pilots in the morning orange juice, Purple Hearts for lunch, a mouthful of Coast-to-Coast for the wee hours of the night, and you'll droop no more. Ladies and gents, the best cure for time and distance is Speed. And we're all familiar with that, aren't we folks? We've all popped a little pep in our day, haven't we? Puts you on top of the world and clears your sinuses to boot. Wire yourself home with a little methamphetamine sulfate, melts in your mind, not in your mouth. No chocolate mess. Step right up and

AWAKE!

get on the ride, pay no heed to that man with the eight-ball eyes! Start with a little propadrine maybe, from the little woman's medicine cabinet? Clear up that stuffy nose? Then work your way up to the full-tilt boogie, twelve-plus grams of Crystal a day! It kind of grows on you, doesn't it, neighbor! Start eating that Sleep and you won't want to eat anything else. You know all about it, don't you, brothers and sisters of the Civilian Band, you've all been on that roller coaster. The only way to fly."

"Now Ryder, you just calm—"

>"Benzedrine, Dexedrine,
>We got the stash!"

he chants like a high-school cheerleader.

>"Another thousand miles
>Before the crash."

"Mr. Moses, you can't—"

>"Coffee and aspirin,
>No-Doz, Meth.
>Spasms, hypertension,
>Narcolepsy, death.
>
>"Alpha, methyl,
>Phenyl too,
>Ethyl-amine's good for you!
>
>"Cause when you're up you're up,
>An when you're down you're down,
>But when you're up behind Crystal
>You're upside down!"

The airwaves crackle with annoyance. Singing on the CB! Sassing their woman, their Sweetpea, with drug talk and four-syllable words!

"—man's crazy—"

"—'s got to go—"

"—FCC ever hears—"

"—fix his wagon—"

"—like to catch—"

"—hophead—"

"—pill-poppin—"

"—weird talkin—"

"—turn him off!"

"Now boys," modulates Sweetpea, cooing soft and smooth, "I'm sure we can talk this whole thing out. Ryder P., honey, whoever you are, you must be runnin out of fuel. I mean you been going at it for days now, flittin round this Innerstate never coming to light. Must be just all out by now, aren't you?"

"I'm going strong, little lady, I got a bottle full of energy left and a thermos of Maxwell House to wash them down with."

"I don't mean that, Mr. Moses, I mean fuel awl. In't your tanks a little low? Must be runnin pert near empty, aren't you?"

"Madam, you have a point."

"Well if you don't fuel up pretty soon, you just gon be out of luck, Mister, they isn't but one more place westbound between here and that Grand Island town. Now I'mo pull in that Bosselman's up ahead, fill this old hog of mine up. Wynch you just join me, I'll buy you a cup of coffee and we'll have us a little chitchat? That truck you got, whatever it is, can't run on no *pills*."

"Madam, it's a date. I got five or six miles to do and then it's Bosselman's for me and Old Paint here. Yes indeedy."

The other channels come alive. Bosselman's, on the westbound, he's coming down! That Sweetpea could talk tears from a statue, an oyster from its shell. Ryder P. Moses in person, hotdamn!

They barrel onto the off-ramp, eastbound and westbound, full tanks and empty, a steady caravan of light bleeding off the main artery, leaving only scattered four-wheelers to carry on. They line up behind the diner in rows, twin stacks belching, all ears.

"This is that Ryder P. Moses, this is that Ryder P. Moses, in the parking lot at Bosselman's. Meet you in the coffee shop, Sweetpea."

Cab doors swing open and they vault down onto the gravel, some kind of reverse Grand Prix start, with men trotting away from their machines to the diner.

AWAKE!

They stampede at the door and mill suspiciously. Is that him, is that him? Faces begin to connect with handles remembered from some previous nighttime break. Hey, there's old Roadrunner, Roadrunner, this is Arkansas Traveler, I known him from before, he ain't it, who's that over there? Overload, you say? You was up on I-29 the other night, north of Council Bluffs, wun't you? What you mean no, I had you on for pert near a half hour! You were where? Who says? Roadrunner, how could you talk to him on Nebraska 83 when I'm talking to him on I-29? Overload, some-body been takin your name in vain. What's that? You modulated with me yesterday from Rawlins? Buddy, I'm out of that Davenport town last evening, I'm westbound. Clutch Cargo, the one and only, always was and always will be. You're kidding! The name-droppin snake! Fellas we got to get to the bottom of this, but quick.

It begins to be clear, as they form into groups of three or four who can vouch for each other, that this Ryder P. Moses works in mysterious ways. That his voice, strained through capacitors and diodes, can pass for any of theirs, that he knows them, handle and style. It's outrageous, it is, it's like stealing mail or wiretapping, like forgery. How long has he gotten away with it, what has he said using their identities, what secrets spilled or discovered? If Ryder P. Moses has been each of them from time to time, what is to stop him from being one of them now? Which old boy among them is running a double life, which has got a glazed look around the eyes, a guilty twitch at the mouth? They file in to find Sweetpea sitting at a booth, alone.

"Boys," she says, "I believe I just been stood up."

They grumble back to their rigs, leaving waitresses with order pads gaping. The civilians in the diner buzz and puzzle—some mass, vigilante threat? Teamster extor-tion? Paramilitary maneuvers? They didn't like the menu? The trucks roar from the Bosselman's abruptly as they came.

On the Interstate again, they hear the story from Axle Sally. Sally broadcasts from the Husky three miles up on the eastbound side. Seems a cattle truck is pulled up by the pumps there, left idling. The boy doesn't see the driver, all he knows is it's pretty ripe, even for a stock-hauler. Something more than the usual cowshit oozing out from the air spaces. He tries to get a look inside but it's hard to get that close with the smell and all, so he grabs a flashlight and plays it around in back. And what do you think he sees? Dead. Dead for some time from the look of them, ribs showing, legs splayed, a heap of bad meat. Between the time it takes the boy to run in to tell Sally till they get back out to the pumps, whoever it was driving the thing has pumped himself twenty gallons and taken a powder. Then comes the call to Sally's radio, put it on my tab, he says. Ryder P. Moses, westbound.

They can smell it in their minds, the men who have run cattle or have had a stock wagon park beside them in the sleeping lot of some truck stop, the thought of it makes them near sick. Crazy. Stone wild crazy.

"Hello there again, friends and neighbors, this is Ryder P. Moses, the Demon of the Dotted Line, the Houdini of the Highways. Hell on eighteen wheels. Sorry if I inconvenienced anybody with the little change of plans there, but fuel oil was going for two cents a gallon cheaper at the Husky, and I never could pass up a bargain. Funny I didn't see any of you folks there, y'ought to be a little sharper with your consumer affairs. These are hard times, people, don't see how you can afford to let that kind of savings go by. I mean us truckers of all people should see the writing on the wall, the bad news in the dollars and cents department. Do we 'Keep America Moving' or don't we? And you know as well as me, there ain't shit moving these days. Poor honest independent don't have a Chinaman's chance, and even Union people are being unsaddled left and right. Hard times, children. Just isn't enough stuff has to get from here to there to keep us in business. Hell, the only way to make it is to carry miscellaneous freight. Get that per-item charge on a full load and you're golden. Miscellaneous—"

(The blue flashers are coming now, zipping by the westbound truckers, sirenless in twos and threes, breaking onto the channel to say don't panic, boys, all we want is the cattle truck. All the trophy we need for tonight is Moses, you just lay back and relax. Oh those Smokies, when they set their minds to a thing they don't hold back, they hump after it full choke and don't spare the horse. Ryder P. Moses, your ass is grass. Smokey the Bear on your case and he will douse your fire. Oh yes.)

"—freight. Miscellaneous freight. Think about it, friends and neighbors, brothers and sisters, think about what exactly it is we haul all over God's creation here, about the goods and what they mean. About what they actually mean to you and me and everyone else in this great and good corporate land of ours. Think of what you're hauling right now. Ambergris for Amarillo? Gaskets for Gary? Oil for Ogalalla, submarines for Schenectady? Veal for Vermillion?"

(The Smokies moving up at nearly a hundred per, a shooting stream in the outside lane, for once allied to the truckers.)

"Tomato for Mankato, manna for Tarzana, stew for Kalamazoo, jerky for Albuquerque. Fruit for Butte."

AWAKE!

(Outdistancing all the legitimate truckers, the Smokies are a blue pulsing in the sky ahead, the whole night on the blink.)

"Boise potatoes for Pittsburgh pots. Scottsbluff sugar for Tampa tea. Forage and fertilizer. Guns and caskets. Bull semen and hamburger. Sweetcorn, soy, stethoscopes and slide rules. Androids and zinnias. But folks, somehow we always come back empty. Come back less than we went. Diminished. It's a law of nature, it is, a law—"

They come upon it at the 375 marker, a convention of Bears flashing around a cattle truck on the shoulder of the road. What looks to be a boy or a very young man spread-eagled against the side of the cab, a half-dozen official hands probing his hidden-regions. The trucks slow, one by one, but there is no room to stop. They roll down their co-pilot windows, but the only smell is the thick electric blue of too many cops in one place.

"You see im? You see im? Just a kid!"

"—prolly stole it in the first place—"

"—gone crazy on drugs—"

"—fuckin hippie or somethin—"

"—got his ass but good—"

"—know who he is?"

"—know his handle?"

"—seen im before?"

"—the end of him, anyhow."

All order and etiquette gone with the excitement, they chew it over among themselves, who he might be, why he went wrong, what they'll do with him. Curiosity, and already a kind of disappointment. That soon it will be all over, all explained, held under the dull light of police classification, made into just some crackpot kid who took a few too many diet pills to help him through the night. It is hard to believe that the pale, skinny boy frisked in their headlights was who kept them turned around for weeks, who pried his way into their nightmares, who haunted the CB and outran the Smokies. That he could be the one who made the hours between Lincoln and Cheyenne melt into suspense and tension, that he could be—

"Ryder P. Moses, westbound on 80. Where are all you people?"

"Who?"

"What?"

"Where?"

"Ryder P. Moses, who else? Out here under that big black sky, all by his lonesome. I sure would preciate some company, Seems like you all dropped out of the running a ways back. Thought I seen some Bear tracks in my rear-view, maybe that's it. Now it's just me an a couple tons of beef. Can't say these steers is much for conversation, though. Nosir, you just can't beat a little palaver with your truckin brothers and sisters on the old CB to pass the time. Do I have a copy out there? Anybody?"

They switch to the channel they agreed on at the Bosselman's, and the word goes on down the line. He's still loose! He's still out there! The strategy is agreed on quickly—silent running. Let him sweat it out alone, talk to himself for a while and haul ass to catch him. It will be a race.

(Coyote, in an empty flatbed, takes the lead.)

"You're probably all wondering why I called you together tonight. Education. I mean to tell you some things you ought to know. Things about life, death, eternity. You know, tricks of the trade. The popular mechanics of the soul. A little exchange of ideas, communication, I-talk-you-listen, right?"

(Up ahead, far ahead, Coyote sees taillights. Taillights moving at least as fast as he, almost eight-five in a strong crosswind. He muscles the clutch and puts the hammer down.)

"Friends, it's all a matter of wheels. Cycles. Clock hand always ends up where it started out, sun always dips back under the cornfield, people always plowed back into the ground. Take this beef chain I'm in on. We haul the semen to stud, the calves to rangeland, the one-year-olds to the feedlot, then to the slaughterhouse the packer the supermarket the corner butcher the table of J. Q. Public. J. Q. scarfs it down, puts a little body in his jizz, pumps a baby a year into the wife till his heart fattens and flops, and next thing you know he's pushing up grass on the lone prayree. You always end up less than what you were. The universe itself is shrinking. In cycles."

(Coyote closes to within a hundred yards. It is a cattle truck. He can smell it through his vent. When he tries to come closer it accelerates over a hundred, back end careening over two lanes. Coyote feels himself losing control, eases up. The cattle truck eases too, keeping a steady hundred yards between them. They settle back to eighty per.)

"Engines. You can grease them, oil them, clean their filters and replace their plugs, recharge them, antifreeze and STP them, treat them like a member of the family, but poppa, the miles take their toll, Time and Distance bring us all to rust. We haul engines from Plant A to Plant B to be seeded in bodies, we haul them to the dealers, buy them and waltz around a couple numbers, then drag them to the scrapyard. Junk City, U.S.A., where they break down into the iron ore of a million years from now. Some cycles take longer than others. Everything in this world is a long fall, a coming to rest, and an engine only affects where the landing will be.

"The cure for Time and Distance is Speed. Did you know that if you could travel at the speed of light you'd never age? That if you went faster than it, you would get younger? Think about that one, friends and neighbors, a cycle reversed. What happens when you reach year zero, egg and tadpole time, and keep speeding along? Do you turn into your parents? Put that in your carburetor and slosh it around."

And on he goes, into Relativity, the relationship of matter and energy, into the theory of the universe as a great Mobius strip, a snake swallowing its own tail. Leaving Coyote far behind, though the hundred yards between stays constant. On he goes, into the life of a cell, gerontology, cryogenics, hibernation theory. Through the seven stages of man and beyond, through the history of aging, the literature of immortality.

(Through Grand Island and Kearney, through Lexington and Cozad and Gothenburg, with Coyote at his heels, through a hundred high-speed miles of physics and biology and lunatic-fringe theology.)

"You can beat them, though, all these cycles. Oh yes, I've found the way. Never stop. If you never stop you can outrun them. It's when you lose your momentum that they get you.

"Take Sleep, the old whore. The seducer of the vital spark. Ever look at yourself in the mirror after Sleep has had hold of you, ever check your face out? Eyes pouched, neck lined, mouth puckered, it's all been worked on, cycled. Aged, Wrinkle City. The cycle catches you napping and carries you off a little closer to the ground. Sleep, ladies, when it has you under, those crows come tiptoeing on your face, sinking their tracks into you. Sleep, gents, you wake from her half stiff with urine, stumble, out to do an old man's aimless, too-yellow pee. It bloats your prostate, pulls your paunch, plugs your ears, and gauzes your eyes. It sucks you, Sleep, sucks you dry and empty, strains the dream from your mind and the life from your body."

(Reflector posts ripping by, engine complaining, the two of them barreling into Nebraska on the far edge of control.)

"And you people let it have you, you surrender with open arms. Not me. Not Ryder P. Moses. I swallow my sleep in capsules and keep one step ahead. Rest not, rust not. Once you break from the cycle, escape that dull gravity, then, people, you travel in a straight line and there is nothing so pure in this world. The Interstate goes on forever and you never have to get off.

"And it's beautiful. Beautiful. The things a sleeper never sees open up to you. The most beautiful dream is the waking one, the one that never ends. From a straight line you see all the cycles going on without you, night fading in and out, the sun's arch, stars forming and shifting in their signs. The night especially, the blacker the better, your headlights making a ghost of color on the roadside, focusing to climb the white line. You feel like you can ride deeper and deeper into it, that night is a state you never cross, but only get closer and closer to its center. And in the daytime there's the static of cornfields, cornfields, cornfields, flat monotony like a hum in your eye, like you're going so fast it seems you're standing still, that the country is a still life on your windshield."

(It begins to weave gently in front of Coyote now, easing to the far right, nicking the shoulder gravel, straightening for a few miles, then drifting left. Nodding. Coyote hangs back a little further, held at bay by a whiff of danger.)

"Do you know what metaphor is, truckin mamas and poppas? Have you ever met with it in your waking hours? Benzedrine, there's a metaphor for you, and a good one. For sleep. It serves the same purpose but makes you understand better, makes everything clear, opens the way to more metaphor. Friends and neighbors, have you ever seen dinosaurs lumbering past you, the road sizzle like a fuse, night drip down like old blood? I have, people, I've seen things only gods and the grandfather stars have seen, I've seen dead men sit in my cab beside me and living ones melt like wax. When you break through the cycle you're beyond the laws of man, beyond CB manners or Smokies' sirens or statutes of limitations. You're beyond the laws of nature, time, gravity, friction, forget them. The only way to win is never to stop. Never to stop. Never to stop."

The sentences are strung out now, a full minute or two between them.

"The only escape from friction is a vacuum."

(Miles flying under, North Platte glowing vaguely ahead on the horizon, Coyote, dogged, hangs on.)

There is an inexplicable crackling on the wire, as if he were growing distant. There is nothing for miles to interfere between them. "The shortest distance between two points—ahh—a straight line."

(Two alone on the plain, tunneling Nebraska darkness.)

"Even the earth—is falling. Even—the sun—is burning out."

AWAKE!

(The side-to-side drifting more pronounced now, returns to the middle more brief. Coyote strains to pick the voice from electric jam. North Platte's display brightens. Miles pass.)

"Straight—"

There is a very loud crackling now, his speaker open but his words hung, a crackling past the Brady exit, past Maxwell. (Coyote creeping up a bit, then lagging as the stock-hauler picks up speed and begins to slalom for real. Coyote tailing it like a hunter after a gut-ripped animal spilling its last, and louder crackling as it lurches, fishtails, and lurches ahead wheels screaming smoke spewing saved only by the straightness of the road and crackling back when Coyote breaks into the Band yelling Wake up! Wake up! Wake up! pulling horn and flicking lights till the truck ahead steadies, straddling half-on half-off the right shoulder in direct line with the upspeeding concrete support of an overpass and he speaks. Calm and clear and direct.)

"This is Ryder P. Moses," he says. "Going west. Good night and happy motoring."

(Coyote swerves through the flameout, fights for the road as the sky begins a rain of beef.)

I MUST KEEP DRIVING NOW
Matthew Roher

My blanket dreams of hurtling snow.
Subway cars come home.
My tunnels start to shimmer
in their black dreams.
I haven't beat myself against sleep.
Two hours at top speed is twenty minutes.
I must keep driving now and just feel dreams
outside. I am an empty obelisk again
still crying at seven, in the sharpened air.
Asleep, her thin minutes love me for an hour.
I've been visited with horrors awake
in a vast black miserable apartment.
I put some thought into it, then I forget.
Everyone dreams he sleeps in his crib.

INSOMNIA
(AS CONVEYED THROUGH ONE MIND'S IRC CHANNEL)
EDWARD CHAMPION

* Now talking in #Insomnia

* Topic is 'Fer the love of Christ, can we get this body to sleep?'

* Set by Morpheus on Thu Jan 26 02:50:21

* Coffee has joined #Insomnia

<ShutEye> what ya do that 4?

* logic has quit IRC (Read error: caffeine from client)

* redbull has joined #Insomnia

<ShutEye> you're going to reduce us to desperate masturbation

<redbull> Well, if we have to wake up in three hours . . .

<Morpheus> youll need sum zees

* panic has joined #Insomnia

<panic> hello out there . . .

<ShutEye> panic? Did you have to come in now?

<panic> We didn't sleep last night either.

<redbull> need more of me? lol!

<Coffee> don't worry, redbull . . .

I got booted last night too when the moderator went to the b-room :)

* BladderKontrol has joined #sex

<BladderKontrol> Hey guys! anyone wana dance?

<ShutEye> not really, but if it gets these lamerz off

<Morpheus> who ya talking about?

<ShutEye> coffee and redbull

<Morpheus> hang on . . .

* Coffee has quit IRC (Flushed through urinary tract)

<Morpheus> is that better?

<ShutEye> killer script, morpheus

\<Morpheus\> i am the god here after all

\<redbull\> still here

\<ShutEye\> damn

* midnightMunchies has joined #Insomnia

\<midnightMunchies\> asl?

\<ShutEye\> you got something to kill the munchies, Morph?

midnightMunchies was kicked by Morpheus (Appetite Suppressant!)

\<redbull\> no problems here . . . i go down better w/o food

Morpheus sets mode: +b ShutEye

\<ShutEye\> Thanks Morph!

* redbull has quit IRC (Drink timeout)

\<Morpheus\> no more caffeine

* drowzy has joined #Insomnia

\<drowzy\> hey gang . . . getting closer

\<Morpheus\> one sec . . .

\<drozy\> I wan*()&*(*(j jkl)*)(*()f_

NO CARRIER

SUNDAY

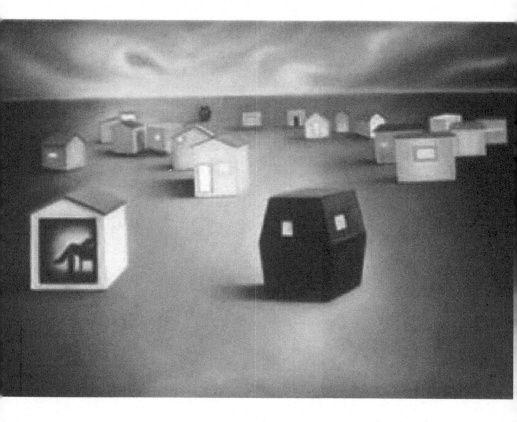

Ice Palace

DEEPLY PSYCHOLOGICAL
REBECCA WOLFF

Heavy with child
up at dawn
I listen and listen to the racket of the birds
but they do not wait for a response
before they ask another question.

So many things seem at an end.
What does not is obvious
and bears no contemplation
or song.

And then I surfaced
a whole matrix
or rubric

magical thinking
other kinds of thinking

but in layers, you understand,

with supremacy
a honeycomb.

FROM THE INSOMNIA DRAWINGS
LOUISE BOURGEOIS

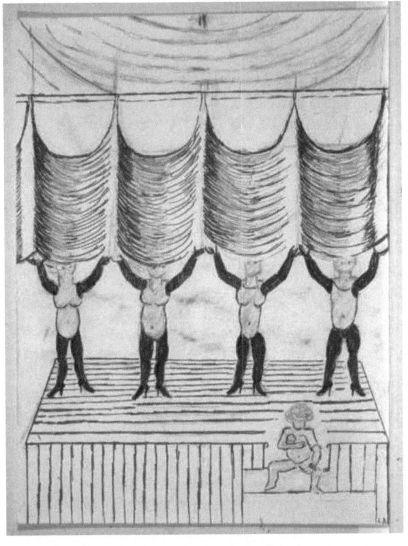

The Insomnia Drawings (detail), 1994-1995
220 mixed media works on paper of varying dimensions
Daros Collection, courtesy Cheim & Read, New York
Photo: Christopher Burke

EAR ON SLUMBER
WILLIAM WALTZ

The body falls gladly
away from the vertical axis
onto shoals of whipped latex
like a beached whale's blubber bundle
dwindles and strands its comical
architecture on golden sands.

After the eyes have sunk
into dark wells like punctured buckets
and fingers have given up their grip,
the bony labyrinth continues its commerce.
When the tongue finally unfurls
and teeth relax, a hammer-anvil tryst

persists: highway hiss, reckless
nighthawk screech, screened whisper of westerlies,
pillowed moan sandwiched between catfights,
clink of the can man, wobble of his wheel
on alley gravel, siren conjuring igneous replies.
Is it possible that this tympan, this trampoline

of cells is all that knows the way back?
A sentinel stands at this threshold and keeps a log
of nocturnal maneuvers whose elements
show up as obscure references the self scribbles.
One of two alarms may sound. We're either too close
to the light or too far from the rocks.

POEM TRYING TO WARM UP ALL ICELAND
Matthew Roher

We are trying to warm up all Iceland
with the local liquor & hot chocolate
& set our feet on fire, still soaking in
the North Sea & I'm breathless far from home.
The little plastic bride, the groom, do not
feel a thing, they will never see the cairn
I built beside the mountain lake. Breathe in,
the air in Husavik smells like Clamato
juice, distinctly of celery & the sea.
Everyone is asleep but the light is on.

I WISH I WERE AN INSOMNIAC
BUD PARR

I used to be an insomniac. I feared going to bed for the tossing and turning, the five a.m. panic of not getting enough sleep to survive the day. The cycle of exhaustion and adrenaline-induced exuberance lasted for nearly a decade and then it went away. Not mysteriously or anything; I got married, changed jobs and I suppose my life expended its daily dose of energy in some way that shortly after I put my head down I opened my eyes to cracks of sunrise through the curtains.

I hated bed for so long before I came to love it. Without the angst of my former sleepless nights, bed became a sanctuary, a lovely place to frolic with my son, read a good book or just lay muscleless and think.

But now the mattress has turned. If I come near the bed I start to feel drowsy. It seems to know what I want, and what I want is sleep.

There's no time for sleep! There are things to do; work, reading, a family life, a social life. But all I can do is sleep. Oh gentle bed! Soft sheets, warm flannel in the winter, crisp and cool in the summer, I love you. Yet I can't have you. I can't afford to spend my nights and days in bed.

I once heard that Edith Wharton spent much of her day writing in bed, casually tossing aside finished manuscript pages for her secretary to type. I visited her restored home in Lenox, Massachusetts, "The Mount," complete with re-created bed, as fluffy and extravagant as you might expect for a woman of her turn-of-the-century wealth. I could only imagine the pleasure that must have been, sprawling paper over the sheets, sunlight washing the room of any hint of the troubled New England winters she so deftly wrote about.

I can only imagine. My Whartonesque attempts at writing in bed—sans secretary—leave my somnambulant fingers working the keyboard of my laptop. Even with the whirring-hot computer on my thighs, my pseudo-narcolepsy seeps in and all those bells and whistles are powerless against the weight of my eyelids.

The real problem is that I work at home and, necessarily, my office is in the bedroom. There's only room for a small desk and chair, and that bed; that damn bed is achingly close. It doesn't matter how much sleep I get at night, all I want is bed and when I'm in the office I can have it any time.

Now I sleep so much that I never have any real need or even desire for it. It's just something that I know I'm going to do; sleep, sleep . . . sleep. Once everyone has left the house in the morning, I'll take a quick nap before answering emails and phone calls. Things slow down around eleven, at which point I take off all my clothes, slip between the covers, pull them over my head and curl up into a deep wondrous sleep through lunch.

No matter how many times I tell myself this is the last nap, I'm back at it again, drooling on my pillow. For a long time my wife didn't know the extent of my habit. She had no idea how I sneak in little naps here and there, how the mere act of extending my foot from my desk chair to the edge of the mattress sends me right to bed, reeling into a dream state where I imagine that all my deadlines are being met, my editors are stunned by my brilliance and my wife is happy with my catapulting career.

When I'm out in the world all I think about is bed. Lately I've found myself going to Macy's and sampling the mattresses there, or going to the Duxiana store and wrapping my arms around one of their impossibly expensive beds with thousands of sturdy Swedish steel springs. The luxury of it all!

But I long for the days of my insomnia. Back then, I was miserable but I was a powerhouse of activity. Sure, some nights I spent confined in the small world of Nickelodeon with little more than a bag of chips and a pint of Breyers for comfort, but I had intensity too. In between the desperation and nagging despair, I wrote like I never have since. Somehow, the inability to think straight from lack of sleep freed my mind of its constraints. The raw nerve of my consciousness was laid bare for me to touch and the result, I have to say, was pure genius.

I developed psoriasis on my hands, perhaps from nervousness, and I drank more coffee than I care to admit. At that time, I did most of my work on a legal pad with pencil and despite my wonderful creativity, I couldn't read any of it as a result of trembling hands and difficulty holding my writing instrument. It's a shame really. All that perfection jettied into obsolescence by the very cause of its creation.

I'd gladly trade my current blissfulness for that miserably productive time, but I'm so happy. I haven't had any decent work in months after missing deadlines and my wife has left for her mother's, but I don't care, I can't care! I'll get back to it. I just need this time, time with my 300 thread-count Egyptian cotton sheets and downy down comforter. Maybe I deserve it after so many years of insomnia. I just want to give myself over to my bed, to block out any sense of myself and the banality of everyday life that I was so acutely aware of when I couldn't sleep.

During my years of insomnia it was a struggle to do anything and everything meant something, even dealing with those lifeless customers at the bank where I worked who wanted nothing more in life than to have their passbook stamped. In bed there are no savings accounts, no bank managers for my aggravation; there's only a world of my making and I don't see how I can give that up.

But alas, I want my family back. I don't really see the problem, why my wife would be so against a little harmless sleep, but I told her I would quit. A friend who understands these things suggested that I try a combination of bee pollen and xanax, a palindrome for a palindromic condition I suppose. This combination, he said, would keep me up and even things out. So that's what I'm doing now. I've taken up coffee again too, but I bought an espresso machine. I created my own drink that I dare any of those Frappuccino types to try. I call it a Cafe Pollenato. Two double shots of espresso—that's four shots altogether—two ounces of hot purified water, a dollop of steamed milk and a bee pollen chaser.

The xanax keeps everything in balance. The tips of my fingers are tingling. It's been three days without bed. It seems to be working. Can you tell? Can you tell? Can you tell?

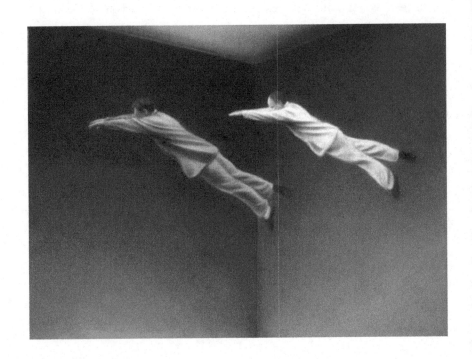

O Sleep

THE PAJAMAIST
MATTHEW ZAPRUDER

In my dream, I was writing a novel called *The Pajamaist*.

There had been a marked advance in the field of suffering. Researchers in the Institute for the Advancement of Reduction of Suffering had discovered it could be transferred, painlessly, from one subject to another. What did this mean in practical terms? No one had to suffer any longer, at least not for free!

We had only to sleep in each others' pajamas, or take some kind of pill to supplement the pajama switching, I hadn't yet dreamed this out.

The first, and greatest of all the sufferers was the Pajamaist, an unemployed white whale in his mid-thirties. I mean male.

When I sleep I don't wear pajamas. I prefer to sleep naked, and thrash the bedsheets around until they wrap me in a protective covering with only my head and feet exposed. Each of my sleeping partners has added to the catalog of possible means of exhibiting displeasure with this nightly process, yet suspiciously, not one has ever thought to buy me pajamas.

Maybe they think pajamas would make me resemble a float in the annual Sleep Parade.

Well there should be.

Once I bought a pair of white silk pajamas, it ended badly.

The Pajamaist had been privately operating as a sufferer, nights and weekends for a few friends and relatives, who in their days and nights began to exhibit such characteristics of a totally suffer-free existence that Researchers from the Institute began to notice weird spikes in their suffer graphs, and hired an Investigator.

The Investigator took the Suffer Location Graphs into the city and began to search for the spike sources, radiating so obviously through their days (and incidentally creating new and additional alienation suffering in the co-workers, wives and ex-girl-friends surrounding them that there is to this day some quiet speculation in the corners that like matter in the universe or total weight within a nuclear family unit suffering has an immutable quotient and can never be reduced, only transferred) that it was easy to trace these rays of suffer-free happiness back from the subjects to their common source, a tiny impossibly black dot of suffering.

Tracing back the suffer location rays to an apartment near the center of the un-named city, the Investigator took a room across the street and watched through black plastic binoculars he had been given on one of his early birthdays so that he could, when taken to the arena, more clearly see the successes of his invincible team, whose name had been recently changed at the insistence of the city fathers.

Sleeping, at first the Pajamaist looked peaceful. Then began the Throes. They were horrible to watch and produced great suffering in the one who was watching. Therefore, instinctively, in order to shield the watcher from further suffering, the Pajamaist isolated himself, a procedure quickly coded as part of the Suffer Transfer Protocol, so as not to merely spread out in a thin at first undetectable but ulti-mately equally palpable over a longer period of time layer, but actually to reduce, the Total Quantity of Suffering in the world. For one can easily see how observing the Throes of the Pajamaist must render in the watcher new suffering, and fail to reduce anything.

Long after the histories of the period had been exhaustively written, a secret mi-nority of revisionists gathered in silence to theorize this self-imposed isolation was in itself the necessary and sufficient key to the Suffer Transfer Protocol. The Pill was totally unnecessary, and one could achieve the same effect in free communities just large enough to permit their own isolation protocols surrounding the general prin-ciple of isolation of the Object. In my dream we lost contact, and believe they were somehow overheard, or eaten.

The Investigator further noted that in the course of his observations (and especially at night when he should have been sleeping) he had divined in the Throes nine varieties of suffering in addition to the tenth, the Purely Physical: suffering because others suffer less than you; suffering because others suffer more than you; suffering because there is suffering at all; suffering for "no reason"; suffering because there can be suffering for "no reason"; suffering because there are logical connections but no god or vice versa; suffering because you have in the past suffered and thus "wasted time"; suffering because you will again in the future suffer and thus "waste time"; and suffering because those you love have, are, or will in the future suffer from any and all of the varieties.

Independently the researchers had come exactly to this Categorization System, but, fearing the Investigator would in his newfound boldness go found a Competing Institute, diagnosed him as borderline schizomniac anal-suppressive and suggested an Eastern Treatment.

Or more accurate, found yet another Competing Institute, for in addition to the Institute for the Advancement of Reduction of Suffering there was the Institute to Speculate on Theories of Suffer Reduction. In this Institute were gathered the ex-girlfriends, mensheviks, priests, standardized testers, and other remnant heirs to the ragtag opposition to the end of the era of randomly allocated suffering, those who both proclaimed and believed that while suffering could not actually be transferred or reduced, one could speculate on the matter, and arrive through the glory of abstract mathematics at a theoretical solution to the "Problem of Suffering."

With the advent of the Pill, the latter Institute began to suffer from a serious lack of funding, and no longer figures in the dream.

The Pill is small and blue, and contains within it one specklet of a substance that cannot without violating certain totally proprietary events be very accurately described. In my dream it was called either the Small Blue, the Small Blue Vehicle, or Pajama's Little Helper.

Wearing the pajamas of a soon-to-be Former Sufferer, by ingesting the Small Blue Vehicle the professional Sufferer is in a secret and as far as the non-profit Institute

AWAKE!

is concerned totally proprietary way open to the suffering of the original sufferer as transferred through physical droplets, night sweats, the essence of palpitations connected directly to the most concentrated form of suffering, in sleep.

True, suffering that occurs in waking is more surprisingly painful, especially in the morning, when a Waker feels mocked and betrayed by the very fact of day. One could very well even call consciousness openness to the possibility of hurt, though one hesitates to light the headlamp and trundle off deeper into that forest of rue.

Nevertheless, the pain of this conscious suffering (which occurs at a time of waking, or relative awareness, or daylight) is in no way correspondent to the *concentration* of suffering, which is at its highest potency during the first hours of sleep. We just think suffering hurts less in sleep because we are sleeping. In our own nightmare throes, we excrete the suffering, and though more exhausted wake purified and ready for day. But an excess of suffering cannot be fully excreted in sleep, and accumulates, accreting.

This, by the way, is why insomniacs, otherwise known as Pure Subjects, have such an aspect of deprivation and suffering, never having a natural opportunity in sleep to excrete it.

I am not, nor have I ever been an insomniac. I sleep like a baby, albeit a very agitated one. I am the eldest of countless children, and therefore received exactly my share of attention, enough to ensure in me from toddlerhood to the present a gentle, non-geometric increase in smile frequency well within melancholia parameters.

It occurs to me now that watching someone else suffer, or even waiting in a different white room designed for Subjects where I could not see the Sufferer but know he suffered for me, would in and of itself constitute suffering, so there would have to arise in my dream some kind of solution. Such a solution could be so horrible that I am tempted to cease thinking of this mechanism any further.

Yet here I can imagine the Pajamaist, suffering quietly and unobserved in his room, asleep in some ways, awake in so many others. I feel for him not suffering, but the kind of pleasurable yet very real sorrow I feel only in my dream life, where the bright colored objects of pre-cognition someone is quietly encouraging me to fit together keep falling from a very high table, and the first words I learn to speak are I'm sorry, I realize this is important to you, but it just seems like a bit too much trouble, this fitting together, and anyway I get confused.

WHO? HOW? HUH?
Contributors' Notes

WHO? Steve Almond is the author, most recently, of *The Evil B.B. Chow & Other Stories* which includes the story "Lincoln, Arisen." For other excerpts of the book and various further perversions, you can check out www.bbchow.com.

HOW? "I've been obsessed with Lincoln for years, as a figure of tremendous moral courage and personal tragedy. He died for the sins of this country, and knew he was going to die, because his dreams told him so. I wanted to set him free from this burden, and I wanted Frederick Douglass there to see him off. Both men deserved fates happier than history imposed on them. The exact opposite, by the way, is true of George W. Bush. He is a man without the character even to remember his nightmares."

WHO? Jonathan Ames is the author of six books, including *Wake Up, Sir!* and *I Love You More Than You Know*.

HOW? "'Insomni-Whack' was originally one of my City Slicker columns for *New York Press* (I wrote this column from 1997-2000), and if I recall correctly, I started the piece after a night of insomnia, recounting the night of sleeplessness up until the recounting of the writing of the first sentence of the piece . . . one of those endings where the writer sits down to write what you've just read . . . that sort of thing."

WHO? Simon Armitage was born in 1963 and lives in West Yorkshire. He has published nine volumes of poetry including *Killing Time* (Faber & Faber, 1999) and *Selected Poems* (Faber & Faber, 2001), and has received numerous awards for his poetry, including the Sunday Times Author of the Year, the Forward Prize and the Lannan Award. He writes for radio, television and film, and is the author of four stage plays and two novels. He also received an Ivor Novello Award and a BAFTA for his song-lyrics in the Channel 4 film *Feltham Sings*. Simon Armitage has taught at the University of Leeds and the University of Iowa's Writers' Workshop, and currently teaches at Manchester Metropolitan University.

AWAKE!

HOW? "Having suffered myself from insomnia, I've always been interested in those waking hours that take on a kind of dreamlike quality, so in the poem I've substituted a dream sequence for what might ostensibly be thought of as a time of sleeplessness. The poem also involves a girl who cannot realize her dreams and a pop star (Ricky Wilson is the lead singer of Leeds band The Kaiser Chiefs) whose dreams have become real. It's also meant to be funny."

WHO? Margaret Atwood is the author of more than forty books of fiction, poetry, and critical essays. Her most recent book *The Tent*, a collection of mini-fictions, was published by Nan A. Talese/Doubleday. Her novel, *Oryx and Crake*, was short-listed for the Man Booker Prize and the Giller Prize in Canada. Her other books include the 2000 Booker Prize winning, *The Blind Assassin*, *Alias Grace*, which won the Giller Prize in Canada and the Premio Mondello in Italy, *The Robber Bride*, *Cat's Eye*, *The Handmaid's Tale* and *The Penelopiad*. Margaret Atwood lives in Toronto with writer Graeme Gibson.

HOW? No comment.

WHO? Nicholson Baker is the author of seven novels, including *The Mezzanine*, *Vox*, *A Box of Matches* and *Checkpoint*. He received the National Book Critics Circle Award in 2001.

HOW? "I lie awake in a float-state and images, often involving spatulas, drift by. One night in May 1986, I thought of a sheep's eyes straining as it pole-vaulted in slow motion over a high bar. I made a note, 'sheep pole-vaulting,' in the back of a paperback and wrote a paragraph about it early the next morning."

WHO? Priscilla Becker's book of poems, *Internal West*, won *The Paris Review's* book prize, and was published in 2002. Her work has appeared in *Open City*, *Fence*, *Raritan* and *The Paris Review*. She teaches writing at Columbia University, and writes music reviews for *Filter* magazine.

HOW? "Because you asked me to."

WHO? Aimee Bender is the author of three books, most recently the story collection *Willful Creatures*. Her fiction has been published in *Granta*, *GQ*, *Harper's*, *The Paris Review*, *Tin House* and more, as well as heard on PRI's "This American Life."

HOW? "This story was a way to explore the idea of balancing things—what happens if a person slept less? What would be the cost? What happens if everything is symmetrical in this person's world? Somehow that was the starting point, and I just tried to follow it from there."

WHO? Gwenda Bond stays up late in Lexington, Kentucky. She posts often about books and writing at her blog, *Shaken & Stirred* (http://gwendabond.typepad. com).

HOW? "When I began thinking about insomnia, I felt superior. I sleep like a just and exhausted baby, puzzling at my friends' up-at-3-a.m. woes. But then I remembered that not sleeping used to be a defining characteristic of my personality. I figured I should write about that."

WHO? Louise Bourgeois (born December 25, 1911, Paris) is an artist and sculptor, whose work has been strongly influenced by surrealism. Her parents were involved in repairing tapestries, although at fifteen she studied mathematics at the Sorbonne. Geometry contributed to her early cubist work in painting and drawing, though she later also studied at the École des Beaux-Arts and worked as an assistant to Fernand Léger. In 1938, she moved with her American husband to New York City, where she continued her studies at the Art Students League. By the 1940s, she had turned her attention to sculptural work, for which she is now recognized as a twentieth-century leader. Louise Bourgeois continues to reside in New York City.

HOW? "In the abstract Insomnia drawings, I talk about the self in relation to others. They come from a deep need to achieve peace, rest and sleep. They come directly from the unconscious. It is a receptive mode. The abstract drawings relate to unconscious memories. The realistic drawings are an overcoming of negative memory, the need to erase, and to get rid of it. These drawings are pinned down in time and location. They rely on the accuracy of memory. Far from sleep inducing, the realistic drawings are problems to be solved. The how to get what you want certainly keeps you up. The more abstract drawings are pleasurable exorcises—the desire to fall asleep, to find peace in rhythm and pattern. Both are indispensable. The more I master the subject and concentrate on the aesthetic, the more pleasure. Anything aesthetic is pleasurable. A realistic drawing excites your curiosity, it does not provoke an aesthetic enjoyment. One is intellectual—a problem to be solved. The other is passive. The enjoyment of the aesthetic is passive. You let yourself be happy—enjoy things."

WHO? Arthur Bradford's first book, *Dogwalker*, was published by Knopf in

2001 and Vintage paperback in 2002. He is the recipient of an O. Henry Award and his fiction has appeared in *Esquire*, *Zoetrope* and *McSweeney's*. He is also the director of the documentary series "How's Your News?" which has appeared on HBO, PBS and Trio.

HOW? "An Irish friend of mine told me once, 'If you ever get stuck writing, just put an Irish guy in the story and then it can go anywhere.' I wasn't really sure what that meant, but I thought I would try it for this story. I didn't really have it planned out. Paul O'Malley is a combination of characters I've known. He's good at heart, just at loose ends. I've noticed that when you go without sleep, things can get kind of batty. I spent a rainy afternoon in Zanesville, Ohio and found it to be a nice town. Dick Cheney was scheduled to visit there the next day, but we left before he arrived."

WHO? Steve Brykman left medical school in his third year to pursue a career writing jokes as Managing Editor of *National Lampoon*. His work has appeared in *Playboy.com*, *Cracked*, *Nerve* and *The New Yorker* where he was featured in Talk of the Town. He has written for or appeared on *Prairie Home Companion*, Comedy Central, G4TV and the Food Network. As a writing fellow at the University of Massachusetts, his fiction was awarded the Harvey Swados prize. Grace Paley called his writing "As good as anything else out there," which is about as high a compliment as he ever hopes to get.

HOW? "I felt sure I had run out of things to write about. But one day on the toilet, the *L.A. Weekly's* back page proved me wrong. Was I 'Anxious?' the page boldly asked. Yes. 'Depressed?' Indubitably. 'Having trouble sleeping?' Without a doubt. Out of these self-realizations, I found the topic for my next book. I would sign up for as many medical research studies as I could find, and subject myself, body and soul, to science for the betterment of society."

WHO? W. Bruce Cameron is a nationally syndicated columnist. He is the author of *How to Remodel a Man* and the bestselling *8 Simple Rules for Dating My Teenage Daughter*, which was turned into a show on ABC. He's an *O Magazine* contributor and has appeared on Oprah.

HOW? "I don't know about everyone else, but I swear my brain talks to me, usually at night, and usually in a most irritating fashion. During the day, when I'm working or driving, my brain pretty much shuts off. I thought it would be interesting for other people to hear what my brain has to say, so I wrote it down during a night of insomnia."

WHO? Edward Champion is a writer in San Francisco. His most recent play, *Wrestling an Alligator*, resulted in at least one death threat. His satirical riffs on books can be experienced at his blog, *Return of the Reluctant* (www.edrants.com).

HOW? "The essay was guided by the steady hand of personal experience, and molded into shape by the more feral elements of curiosity and information collection. I am not certain if it offers a complete remedy, but for those who find their circadian rhythms triggered by similar stimuli, it is my firm duty to reassure you that you are not alone."

WHO? Born in 1962, Claro has written eight novels—most recently, *Electric Flesh*, published in 2006 by Soft Skull Press—and has translated many American writers (Pynchon, Vollmann, Brian Evenson, Dennis Cooper, etc.). He lives in Paris with his wife, film-director Marion Laine, and their four children.

HOW? "Why should sleeping be only a human activity? Obviously, things know some rest, quiet and mute as they are. On the other hand, maybe they don't sleep so well. Maybe they're troubled."

WHO? Joshua Cohen was born in Southern New Jersey in 1980. He is the author of *The Quorum* (Twisted Spoon Press, 2005) and *Cadenza for the Schneidermann Violin Concerto* (Fugue State Press, 2006). He lives in New York City.

HOW? "I came to write 'On Getting the Sheets to Stay On the Bed . . .' one night in bed, reading the book of Genesis. The Biblical waters above and the waters below became sheets, refusing to become tamed to the bed. I went to my desk, at which I wrote this piece and fell asleep."

WHO? Karen Condon earned an MFA from the University of Massachusetts in Amherst in 1993. While at UMass, she was the recipient of an Associated Writing Programs Intro Award and The Harvey Swados Award for Fiction. She has had short stories published in *Bottomfish Magazine*, *Kansas Quarterly*, *Arkansas Review*, *Antigonish Review* and *Sonora Review*. In 2004, she was a finalist in the Massachusetts Cultural Council Artist Grants Competition. She recently completed a novel, and has begun another.

HOW? "As a captionist for deaf college students, I occasionally find myself working in classes with rather foreign subject matter—such as the chemistry class I witnessed last summer. 'Periodic Table' is the result of that experience."

WHO? Howard Cruse's underground comic book stories began appearing in the early '70s. In 1983, he launched Wendel, a comic strip that was featured in The Advocate during much of the subsequent decade. His critically acclaimed graphic novel Stuck Rubber Baby was published in 1995 and in 2000 Olmstead Press issued Wendel All Together, a compilation of the entire Wendel series from beginning to end. Cruse's most recent book, the cartoonist's illustrated adaptation of a fable by Jeanne E. Shaffer entitled The Swimmer With a Rope In His Teeth, was published by Prometheus Books in 2004. Visits to Cruse's comics-packed web site Howard Cruse Central (www.howardcruse.com) are encouraged.

HOW? "'A Little Night Misery' is very personal to me, being a fictionalized burlesque of one of the numerous long, dark nights of self-doubt I endured after moving from Alabama to New York City in 1977. The story stands in for the painting generated by Headrack's imagined death splotch on the sidewalk: art that surprises the artist by flowering out of despair."

WHO? A. Roger Ekirch, a professor of history at Virginia Tech, is the author of At Day's Close: Night in Times Past. Previous publications include Poor Carolina: Politics and Society in Colonial North Carolina, 1729–1776 (1981) and Bound for America: The Transportation of British Convicts to the Colonies, 1718–1775 (1987).

HOW? "I became interested in the historical nature of sleep a during the course of working on my recent book, At Day's Close: Night In Times Past. My enthusiasm for the subject grew with the recognition that pre-industrial households went to enormous lengths to ensure both the tranquility and the safety of their slumber. Still more intriguing, as I discovered, was the pattern of segmented sleep that began to emerge from diaries, letters and imaginative literature—references to a first and a second sleep, phrased in such a way as if the prospect of awakening in the dead of the night was perfectly natural."

WHO? Brian Evenson is the author of seven books of fiction, most recently The Open Curtain, which was published by Coffee House Press in 2006. He directs the Literary Arts Program at Brown University.

HOW? "I've been playing around a lot in my fiction lately with notions of story form, so this story starts somewhat humorously and gets more and more serious and despairing. It borrows an 18th-century trick and deliberately 'withdraws' at a certain point, but I think what I'm doing formally gets something across about insomnia in several different ways, about how it feels (at least for me) when you've gone many nights struggling to sleep and have begun to believe you might never sleep again."

WHO? Myles Gordon is a writer/television producer living in Newton, Massachusetts. A past recipient of the Grolier Poetry Prize, he has had poems published in several literary journals, including *Evansville Review, California Quarterly, Chiron Review* and *Spoon River Poetry Review*.

HOW? "I wrote the poem in the midst of coming to terms with a colicky infant and living in a constant state of sleep-deprived euphoria during which I got this grandiose idea that not just the gods and goddesses, but all of us have our own personal mythologies complete with constellations no less stellar than the Olympian ones. As I began to get more sleep, the idea kinda faded—but at least I got this poem and a couple of others from the notion."

WHO? Rose Gowen's stories have recently appeared in *Opium Magazine* and in *Bullfight Review*. She has also been published in the *American Poetry Review, Night Train, Bridge, Kitchen Sink*, and *Pindeldyboz*, and links to her work on the web can be found at www.rosegowen. com. Her short play was produced at Empire Fulton Ferry State Park, in Brooklyn, in the summer of '03, as part of *10 Stories: A Humble Offering to the Manhattan Skyline*.

HOW? "In my poem, I was trying to capture the monotony, as well as the frustration and racing mind of insomnia."

WHO? Franklin H. Head may in fact be no one. According to a "transcbiber's note" that precedes the essay, "The following is a literary hoax, and the letters quoted below are false." The letters in question—which appear in the second section of the essay (unprinted here)—also point to money worries as the cause of Shakespeare's insomnia. They are written by, among others, a "Queer Street" pawnbroker, a lawyer for a litigious actor and a certain Moredcai Shylock, who claims that he would "gladly meet [Shakespeare's] needs [for a loan] at a moderate usance, not more than twenty-five in the hundred."

HOW? That is the question.

WHO? Bob Hicok's fifth collection, *This Clumsy Living*, was published by Pitt earlier this year. His last book was *Insomnia Diary* (Pitt, 2004). He teaches at Virginia Tech and his hobby is stacking boxes.

HOW? "I don't have anything to say about the poems."

WHO? Michael Koenig has published short stories and poetry in *The Cape Rock, Pacific Coast Journal, Poetry: USA, Night Songs* and *Elysian Fields Quarterly*. He reads regularly around the San Francisco Bay Area and is currently working on a collection of short stories about celebrity.

HOW? "The original idea for 'The Man Who Never Sleeps' came from personal research—I got mugged. Over the next few weeks, I wrote about what had happened to me and my lingering dread of walking the streets that I traveled every day. I tried to insert the material I'd written about the mugging into every story I wrote, but it never seemed to fit. As the years passed, I became fascinated by the ways in which reality television magnifies our afflictions and turns them into a kind of performance. I began writing the story in interview form primarily to condense the action into a limited space, but soon the interviewer developed into his own character, mildly venal, but mostly kind. As a former Journalism major, I have felt the same embarrassment that he feels. Why am I asking these rude questions? What gives me the right?"

WHO? Molly Kottemann was born in 1983, the product of a poet and a professor of Decision Sciences. Accordingly, she now splits her time between writing and science, occasionally melding the two. She received her BS in Molecular/Cellular Biology & Genetics from the University of Maryland College Park in 2000, and is currently a fourth-year Ph.D. student in Genetics at Yale University, where she researches cancer and DNA repair.

HOW? "A chronic insomniac, I have long been fascinated by the molecular mechanisms that form the scaffolding of my sleeplessness. My work as a researcher has inculcated in me the desire always to ask not only why, but also how. Even in the throes of exhausted consciousness, I want to tease out the scientific underpinnings, and to translate sometimes pedantic papers on the topic into a more dreamy prose."

WHO? Catie Lazarus is a comedian. Her drivel appears in *The New York Times, Time Out New York, The Forward* and *Heeb Magazine*, where she is an editor. Emerging Comics of New York recently awarded her "Best Comedy Writer." Her website: www.lazarusrising.com

HOW? "I am constantly suffering from sleeping at the wrong hours, meaning I fall asleep when I am supposed to be pushing paper around at a job and then stay up at night. Now, when I stay up late, I am not exactly rewriting the corporate tax code or doing something otherwise useful. I have slept under many desks at way too many day jobs."

WHO? Dubbed "The Thinking Man's Guitar Hero" by *The New Yorker*, Gary Lucas tours the world relentlessly both solo and with several different ensembles, including his longtime band Gods and Monsters, which once counted among its ranks the late singer Jeff Buckley (Lucas co-wrote two of Buckley's most famous hits, "Grace" and "Mojo Pin") and was recently described as "a 21st century Cream" by Rolling Stone. A graduate of Yale University, where he was a DJ and served as Music Director at WYBC FM, Gary's childhood dream of joining Captain Beefheart's Magic Band came true when he recorded two Beefheart albums in the early 80s, *Doc at the Radar Station* (1980) and *Ice Cream for Crow* (1982). Over the course of his career he has recorded everything from Chinese pop to Jewish children's songs to psychedelic rock, and has worked with a range of talents, including, Leonard Bernstein, Lou Reed, Joan Osborne, David Johansen, John Zorn, Peter Stampfel, Kate and Anna McGarrigle and Iggy Pop

HOW? "I came to write 'Me and the Golem' several years ago on commission by the editor of a projected anthology of science and fantasy short stories with Jewish mystical and Kaballistic themes. That particular anthology never did come to life, but I was happy to put my tale in a state of suspended animation for many years, only to wave my hands over it, mutter a few Kabbalistic incantations and reanimate it, Golem-like, for this particular insomnia-themed collection—'To sleep, perchance to dream ... Ay, there's the rub' ... the nocturnal condition of dwelling happily in the arms of Morpheus eludes me frequently in my hop-scotching 'round the world

AWAKE!
in search of audiences for my music/unknown pleasures . . . and I must confess to the downing of an Ambien at 4 a.m. this morning here in Melbourne in order to try and shake off the effects of twenty-five hours by jet from NYC in order to play *The Golem* in a more or less *compos mentis* condition (I'm opening two Australian Festivals of Jewish Cinema here in Melbourne and in Sydney with *The Golem*)."

WHO? Lydia Lunch has been confronting the paying public for three decades, utilizing a variety of media to unleash her inner demons. She began her career by founding the No Wave band Teenage Jesus and the Jerks and later collaborated in film, music and spoken word with Kim Gordon, Thurston Moore, Robert Quine, Excene Cervenka and Hubert Selby, Jr. among many others.

HOW? "'Illusive Bitch' was written under a generous twenty-three-hour deadline granted by the editor as a test to just how little sleep the author could once again survive on. Thanks Pal."

WHO? Jonathan Messinger's work has previously appeared in *Bridge, The Chicago Reader, Rainbow Curve, McSweeney's online, THE2NDHAND* and numerous other publications. Editor of *THISisGRAND*, an online journal of creative non-fiction detailing life on Chicago's public transportation system, he is also the books editor for *Time Out Chicago*.

HOW? "This story was originally written for a reading series I run called The Dollar Store."

WHO? Mark Jay Mirsky founded the magazine *Fiction* in 1972 with Donald Barthelme, Max and Marianne Frisch and Jane De Lynn. A graduate of Harvard College, and Stanford University (M.A.), his first novel *Thou Worm Jacob* was published in 1967 by Macmillan, followed by *Proceedings of the Rabble* and *Blue Hill Avenue* at Bobbs Merrill. A collection of novellas, *The Secret Table* followed in the mid 1970's, and the novel, *The Red Adam* in 1990. In addition he has published several books that mingle the fantastic and the factual, testing the borders of the academic, *My Search for the Messiah, The Absent Shakespeare* and his latest, *Dante, Eros and Kabbalah* (Syracuse University Press.) He is the editor of the *Diaries of Robert Musil* and co-editor of the anthology *Rabbinic Fantasies*.

HOW: Insomnia is one of the conditions of a writer's life. Pushed from the covers or unable to sleep, one floats in a world where time, and therefore space as we now understand, begins to bend and suggest other dimensions. Writers dream of creating realities through words, and so their characters do so, though always expressing the pain of the disjunction. There is no crueler portrait of love in the history of literature than the courtship of Dulcinea by Don Quixote—what a bitter reflection by Cervantes on the the hopeless passion of Catholic Spain. In my case, however, reality almost answered my call, and let me penetrate the image which emerged from the screen whose virtual reality heralds a new religious era.

WHO? C.O. Moed was born on New York's Lower East Side when it was still a tough neighborhood. With a Masters in Dramatic Writing (NYU) and Media Arts / Directing (City College), she was nominated for a Rockefeller Media Arts Fellowship in 2003 and attended the Berlinale Talent Campus and Berlin Today Award Summer Campus 2005. With her partner, filmmaker Ruben Guzman, she writes, shoots and works a day job in NYC.

HOW? "'How Insomnia Saved my Life Until the Night It Tried uo Kill Me' was my attempt to understand the last thirty years of sleeplessness and Stephen Sondheim's repertoire."

WHO? Nicholas Montemarano is the author of the short-story collection *If the Sky Falls* (LSU, 2005) and the novel *A Fine Place* (Context Books, 2002). His fiction has been published in *Esquire, Zoetrope, Agni, Fence, The Pushcart Prize 2003* and many other publications. The recipient of fellowships from the National Endowment for the Arts, The MacDowell Colony and Yaddo, he teaches at Franklin & Marshall College.

HOW? "This story began when I read about an all-girl band in Germany called Hello Bob Ross Superstar after the late feel-good painting instructor. I'm not sure if that's true, but it doesn't matter because it sounds like it could be true. I'm fairly certain there is no such Japanese all-girl punk rock band called Hello Randy Gardner Superstar, though perhaps there should be. There *is* a Randy Gardner who, last time I checked, held the world record for longest amount of time without sleeping: eleven days. He achieved this distinction in 1964 in San Diego at the age of seventeen. A few years ago, a man in Queens named David Axelrod tried to break Gardner's record. The details about his attempt are murky at best, but the short of it is this: he believed he had broken the record, but he really hadn't. I'm not sure if he couldn't properly document his 265 hours awake, or if in his sleep-deprived delirium he miscounted, but

AWAKE!

Randy Gardner's name will remain in the record books, for now. Axelrod committed suicide a few weeks after his failed attempt—he jumped off the Verrazano-Narrows Bridge (of *Saturday Night Fever* fame). When I read about the German band Hello Bob Ross Superstar, something clicked in my brain, and I remembered having read about David Axelrod. There's a connection there. Something about fame—the desire for celebrity, even if small-time celebrity."

WHO? Joyce Carol Oates is the author of the forthcoming novel *The Gravedigger's Daughter*. She is a recipient of the National Book Award and the PEN/ Malamud Award for Excellence in Short Fiction. She is also the recipient of the 2005 Prix Femina for *The Falls*. She is the Roger S. Berlind Distinguished Professor of the Humanities at Princeton University, and she has been a member of the American Academy of Arts and Letters since 1978.

HOW? No comment.

WHO? Robin Palanker is a visual artist living in Culver City, California. Her artwork has been exhibited and collected nationally, and to enhance its "motion-centric" elements, she often uses performing artists as models. In addition to painting, Palanker produced and directed the award winning play *Nijinsky Speaks* and, recently, she received the Sharon Disney Lund Master Teacher Award for her work with gifted high school artists. She wishes that this book had been printed in color.

HOW? "For my 2003 solo show, *Sleep Won't Come*—which was also the inspiration for jazz trumpeter John McNeil's 2004 CD of the same name—I visualized a lifetime of sleeplessness. I am grateful for all those extra hours."

WHO? Bud Parr is a writer and web consultant living and working in Brooklyn, New York with his wife Lynn and young son, Auden. He writes and edits the literary weblog, *Chekhov's Mistress*. This is his publishing debut.

HOW? "My relationship with bed has always been uneasy, first with extended insomnia, now with a desire to have more waking-hours in the day. 'I Wish I Were An Insomniac' arose from that tension."

WHO? Neal Pollack is the author of several books of satirical fiction and a memoir called *Alternadad*. He lives in Los Angeles with his wife Regina and their son Elijah, who wakes up way too early.

HOW? "It's no struggle for me to always pump up the value of sleeping in. I feel that too many adults disdain the experience, and more by choice than you think. A good night's sleep is the healthiest thing in the world."

WHO? Matthew Rohrer is the author of four books of poems: *A Hummock In The Malookas*, which won the 1994 National Poetry Series and was chosen by *Publishers Weekly* as a "Best Book of the Year" for 1995; *A Green Light*, which was shortlisted for the 2005 Griffin Prize; *Satellite*, and *Nice Hat*. In addition, Rohrer collaboratively wrote *Thanks* with Joshua Beckman (an audio CD, *Adventures While Preaching The Gospel Of Beauty*, collects some of their live, improvised collaborative poems from their extensive tour to support the book). Rohrer's poems have appeared in many journals here and overseas, and have been widely anthologized.

HOW? "I wrote the poems in bed, where I write all my poems. I'm a stay at home dad, and don't have much time to write until my son goes to bed. Then I go to bed. Then I realize that I should be writing. So I write in bed. I've been doing this for several years now and now I can't write sitting up, I have to be lying down. Andre Breton said 'poetry should be made in bed, like love.'"

WHO? Davy Rothbart is an author, filmmaker and contributor to *This American Life*, and the editor/publisher of *FOUND Magazine*. His short story collection, *The Lone Surfer of Montana, Kansas*, was published by Simon & Schuster in 2005, and his documentary film *How We Survive* (about the punk band Rise Against) was released by Geffen Records on the DVD *Generation Lost* in 2006.

HOW? "My favorite aspect of going on the road on our *FOUND Magazine* tours is all the amazing finds that folks bring to us at our shows. In San Francisco, a woman presented me with these three mysterious faxes that had appeared one morning in her office fax machine."

WHO? John Sayles is the author of the novels *Pride of the Bimbos*, *Union Dues* and *Los Gusanos*, and the short story collections *The Anarchist's Convention* and *Dillinger in Hollywood*, all published by Nation Books. He is also the writer and director of the films *Return of the Secaucus 7*, *The Brother from Another Planet*, *Lone Star* and many others.

HOW? "I got the idea for the 'I-80 Nebraska' while hitchhiking across the country in the late '60's, getting rides from truckers who needed me to help them stay awake without hallucinating. A few years later the CB (Citizens' Band) radio came on and they were less likely to need the entertainment, although many were still not sleeping for days at a time."

WHO? Charles Simic is a poet, essayist and translator. He has published twenty collections of his own poetry, five books of essays, a memoir and numerous of books of translations. He has received many literary awards for his poems and his translations, including the Pulitzer Prize, the Griffin Prize and the MacArthur Fellowship. *Voice at 3 A.M.*, a volume of his selected later and new poems, was published by Harcourt in 2003 and a new book of poems *My Noiseless Entourage* in the spring of 2005.

HOW? "I have no idea how I wrote 'Hotel Insomnia,' but since I have been a lifelong insomniac who has written many poems about being sleepless, it's easy to guess. Most likely, one day I just recalled my sleepless nights in the years 1958-1959 at Hotel Washington on Washington Place in New York."

WHO? Frank Stack says, "I was born and raised in Texas, well south of Dallas, Houston, Corpus Christi, west Texas and Austin; art degree from U of Texas at Austin, where I formed most of my attitudes. Austin is NOT a Right Wing town. Married in 1959 and, with my wife Robbie, spent several years going from place to place, including school (Art Institute of Chicago, University of Wyoming) and the army (California and Manhattan). Involved with early years of underground cartoons. Taught at University of Missouri, Columbia, from 1963 to retirement in 2002—painting, drawing and even a course in comic strips. Published comics include *New Adventures of Jesus, Amazons, Dorman's Doggie, Feelgood Funnies, Naked Glory* and lots of contributions to other magazines, including *Zero-Zero, Snarf, Rip Off Magazine, National Lampoon, Village Voice* and *American Splendor*."

HOW? "Sleep, dreams, anxiety and over-active imaginative activity during sleep or illness, has always interested me, though it seems to be a fact that I have never really suffered from an inability to sleep at night. But I never could do all-nighters either. One of the reasons we can't really trust our minds, is that the brain in semi-conscious state produces such convincing similitudes of reality, almost exactly like real experience, and our conscious minds are capable of being deceived. I've noticed when I get sleepy while reading that I sometimes close my eyes and think that I am still reading, and will manufacture in my brain long passages that seem to be the same as the book. Then I will wake up and realize that I haven't been reading at all. The sleep stage, I believe, gives rise to hallucinatory experiences, especially if, enhanced by drugs or illness. The comic was, of course, just a joke, making reference first to the idea that it's easy to sleep if there's nothing stirring up your mind. But there's almost always something on your mind to disturb peaceful sleep."

WHO? Susan Steinberg is the author of the story collections *The End of Free Love* and *Hydroplane*. Her stories have appeared or are forthcoming in *Conjunctions*, *Boulevard*, *The Gettysburg Review*, *McSweeney's* and elsewhere. She teaches at the University of San Francisco and is the fiction editor of *Pleiades*.

HOW? "After a night of no sleep, of just lying, sweating in this devastating summer heat in an attic apartment, I poured a glass of water and walked to the window. Now I can't remember if I dropped the glass to the sidewalk or if I just imagined dropping it. I can't remember if I took an aspirin. I know I was in Massachusetts, not Maryland. And at some point, still morning, still in an insomniacal haze, I went into the other room to attempt to write, and eventually it became this story."

WHO? Darin Strauss is the international bestselling author of the award-winning novels *Chang and Eng* and *The Real McCoy*. His work has been translated into thirteen languages and published in seventeen countries. He is currently writing the screenplay to *Chang and Eng* with Gary Oldman. His third novel *The Pursuit of Happiness* will be published by Dutton in 2008.

HOW? "I usually try to avoid sex scenes; they're often cheesy, and what can you do in writing them but titillate the reader? But when I worked on my first novel, *Chang & Eng,* the story of the first famous conjoined twins—who had twenty-one kids between them—I knew I'd have to show the reader how these guys (and their wives) did it. (Whenever I told people what my book was about, that was the first question they asked.) And so, I thought about how weird and funny and awkward it would have been to try getting sleep if you were attached to someone who was losing his virginity. I thought of it as a kind of metaphor for my own insomnia; whenever I personally couldn't sleep, it seemed that something really awful was keeping me awake; what was happening to my character was the manifestation of that predicament—it was sort of the elbows and knees of insomnia. Anyway, that's how I related to the situation of my characters, whose lives were so different from my own."

AWAKE!

WHO? Cricket Suicide is a native Torontonian. In March 2004, she relocated to Los Angeles to pursue her art and music. As someone living with generalized anxiety disorder, she frequently experiences bouts of insomnia. She copes with these by translating them into art.

HOW? "These photos came about during a period of high anxiety for me. A lot had recently changed in my life, I never slept, I only worried, and so one night I decided to document it. It was a therapeutic solution . . . to another sleepless night."

WHO? James Tate was born in Kansas City, Missouri, in 1943. He is the author of numerous books of poetry, including *Worshipful Company of Fletchers* (1994), which won the National Book Award, *Selected Poems* (1991), which won the Pulitzer Prize and the William Carlos Williams Award, and *The Lost Pilot* (1967), which was selected by Dudley Fitts for the Yale Series of Younger Poets. He has also published a novel, *Lucky Darryl* (1977), and a collection of short stories, *Hottentot Ossuary* (1974), and he edited *The Best American Poetry 1997*. His honors include a National Institute of Arts and Letters Award for Poetry, the Wallace Stevens Award and fellowships from the Guggenheim Foundation and the National Endowment for the Arts. He teaches at the University of Massachusetts in Amherst and is currently a Chancellor of The Academy of American Poets.

HOW? "'Red Dirt' reminds me of how we all live, something immense and terrifying buried beneath us."

WHO? Lynne Tillman's book, *This Is Not It*, a collection of twenty-three stories and novellas written in response to twenty-two contemporary artists' work, was published by DAP in 2002. Her most recent novel, *American Genius, A Comedy*, was published by Soft Skull Press in 2006.

HOW? "I was asked to contribute a story to a limited edition photography magazine, published by a French group called Coromandel Press. Their project for the issue was Le Dormir/Sleep, and all of the photographs and stories in it were to be devoted to the idea of sleep. So, voilà, 'Dead Sleep.'"

WHO? William Waltz grew up in Wapakoneta, Ohio, home of the first man on the moon. *Zoo Music*, his first book, was selected by Dean Young as the winner of the Second Annual Slope Editions Book Prize. His poems have appeared in *Denver Quarterly, Exquisite Corpse, Forklift Ohio, Insurance, LIT, Poetry East, Spinning*

Jenny and *Verse*. Waltz is the editor of *Conduit*. He lives in Minneapolis with his wife Brett Astor and their daughter Clark Mercy.

HOW? "When the fear of no sleep vanquishes actual sleep, my mind will often run through a maze of unrelated topics before settling on one, which is examined, disassembled, re-examined and finally reassembled, however askew. Anything could be the subject of such a battery, including, as in this poem, what we hear when we sleep."

WHO? Joe Wenderoth grew up in and around Baltimore. Wesleyan University Press published his first two books of poetry: *Disfortune* (1995) and *It Is If I Speak* (2000). *Letters to Wendy's*, a novel in verse, and *The Holy Spirit of Life: Essays Written for John Ashcroft's Secret Self*, were published by Verse Press in 2000 and 2005 respectively. *No Real Light* was published by Wave Books earlier this year. Wenderoth is Associate Professor of English and teaches in the graduate Creative Writing Program at the University of California, Davis.

HOW? "How I came to write *Letters to Wendy's*: I found a card that said 'Tell Us About Your Visit!'"

WHO? Shannon Wheeler is the recipient of multiple awards, including the Hatch Broadcasting Award (for a Converse tennis shoe commercial) and an Eisner Award (frequently called the Oscar of comics). He started cartooning in the late '80s while studying architecture at UC Berkeley. He has worked in animation and illustration, and has also published a humor magazine for a number of years. *Too Much Coffee Man*, as a comic, has appeared internationally in newspapers, magazines and comic books. Dark Horse Comics has published four graphic novels that collect most of the work. Last year, Wheeler's *Too Much Coffee Man Opera*, co-written with Damian Wilcox and Daniel Steven Crafts, premiered in Portland, Oregon's Brunish Hall.

HOW? "That story has been in my mind for a while. It felt good to get it out. The guy that got me to destroy my model was killed a couple years back. I think about him every now and again. It was good to put him in a story."

WHO? Dara Wier's tenth book, *Remnants of Hannah*, was published last year by Wave Books. Her previous collection, *Reverse Rapture*, appeared from Verse Press in 2005. She directs the MFA program for poets and writers at the University of Massachusetts in Amherst. National Endowment for the Arts, Guggenheim

Foundation and Massachusetts Cultural Council fellowships have supported her work.

HOW? "Beginning sometime in late June [2005], I turned to writing fourteen-line poems as a correction after having written the long poem *Reverse Rapture.* I tried correcting, by which I mean seeking another course, another means, by writing prose through the spring, which I enjoyed, though it didn't really solve the problem of writing poems unrelated to *Reverse Rapture.* Finally circumstances of grief and loss and upheaval conspired to deliver a tone and a means of address such as you see in the poem I sent. There are around fifeen or maybe sixteen of these sort and maybe more, am unsure. Insomnia's unreality profoundly refracts, its moods are never light, never giddy or sweet or hopeful or of any comfort. Insomnia feels most often like a sentence one is waiting to end, doing time in the lonely precincts of unsleeping. Have you ever heard of two people having insomnia together? Well, I guess anything's possible though I suspect each one experiences insomnia alone."

WHO? Rebecca Wolff is the author of two books of poems, *Manderley* (University of Illinois Press, 2001) and *Figment?* (W.W. Norton, 2004). She is the founding editor of the literary journal *Fence* and of its publishing arm, Fence Books. Born and raised in New York City, she has relocated up the Hudson River with her husband, the novelist Ira Sher, and their two children, Asher and Margot.

HOW? "I don't really have any kind of explanation for these poems, sadly; they just were born. Sorry to be so mystical about it, but that's really the way things go around here."

WHO? Beth Woodcome won the 2003 Grolier Prize and has been published in *Gulf Coast, Columbia Journal of Art & Literature* and *Ploughshares* in their Emerging Writers issue. She holds an MFA from Bennington College and currently lives in Cambridge, MA where she is poetry editor of *Agni.*

HOW? "I find that I suffer from insomnia during times of great stress or heartbreak. When writing this I was at the beginning of the end of a relationship. I would spend my nights sorting through memories, and often the simplest experiences from the past were the most painful and the most profound. There are very few things I find more frustrating in my personal life than the loss of love and loss of sleep. Each can be agonizing, feed into the other, and can create the most base, animalistic feelings I've ever experienced."

WHO? Franz Wright's book, *Walking to Martha's Vineyard*, received the 2004 Pulitzer Prize for poetry; his last collection, *God's Silence*, was published by Knopf in 2006. Other available titles include *The Beforelife* and *Ill Lit: Selected & New Poems*. He lives in Waltham, Massachusetts, and is a volunteer facilitator at The Center For Grieving Children.

HOW? "I really don't know what to say about the composition of this particular piece. Sometimes a poem is about the last thing one expects to happen. This one appeared and introduced itself to me, as poems do once in a while—they don't all take years to write—at about 3 a.m. one summer night like an old friend I'd never expected to see again. (Only no one else could see her.) (But then no one else was there to see her—no one ever is, and she doesn't stay very long. You'll have to take my word for it. Well, I suppose nobody has to take my word for anything, what do I care?)"

WHO? Matthew Zapruder is the author of *American Linden*, winner of the Tupelo Press Editor's Prize, and of *The Pajamaist*, published by Copper Canyon in 2006. His book of translations from the Romanian, *Secret Weapon: The Late Poems of Eugen Jebeleanu*, will be published by Coffee House in 2008.

HOW? "The first and only time I have ever woken up laughing was from a dream in which my dream self 'wrote' an entire novel called *The Pajamaist*. In the novel, a tragic hero accidentally discovers a process for transferring suffering. I tried to remember the plot, and to discover for myself the circumstances that would have led to such a discovery. I have little doubt this attempt is the closest I will ever come to writing fiction."

CREDITS

"Lincoln Arisen," by Steve Almond, originally appeared in *The Evil B.B. Chow and Other Stories*, published by Algonquin Books in 2005.

"Insomni-Whack," by Jonathan Ames, appears in the collection *What's Not to Love? The Adventures of a Mildly Perverted Young Writer*, which was published by Vintage Books in 2000.

"In the Secular Night," by Margaret Atwood, was originally published in *Morning in the Burned House* (McClelland & Stewart, Houghton Mifflin, Virago, 1995).

The Mezzanine, by Nicholson Baker, was originally published by Vintage in 1988.

The Insomnia Drawings, 1994-1995, is a series of 220 mixed media works on paper of varying dimensions. It is housed in the Daros Collection and reprinted compliments of Cheim & Read, New York. Photo: Christopher Burke.

"A Little Night Misery," by Howard Cruse, originally appeared in *Barefootz Funnies #3*, published in 1979 by Kitchen Sink Press.

"Dreams Deferred," by A. Roger Ekirch, originally appeared in the Op/Ed section of the *New York Times* on February 19, 2006.

"Shakespeare's Insomnia and the Causes Thereof," by Franklin H. Head, is described as a "literary hoax" published in 1886, though it appears not to have been published until 2001 by Project Guttenberg.

"In the Insomniac Night," by Joyce Carol Oates, originally appeared in the anthology *Black Swan, White Raven*, edited by Ellen Datlow and Terri Windling and published by Avon in 1997.

"I-80 Nebraska, M.490—M.205," by John Sayles, originally appeared in the *Atlantic Monthly* in 1975.

"Hotel Insomnia," by Charles Simic, originally appeared in *Hotel Insomnia*, published by Harvest Books in 1992.

Chang and Eng, by Darin Strauss, was originally published by Dutton in 2000.

"Red Dirt," by James Tate, originally appeared in *Return to the City of White Donkeys*, originally published by Harper Collins in 2005.

"Dead Sleep," by Lynne Tillman, originally appeared in *This Is Not It*, published by Distributed Art Publishers, 2002.

Letters to Wendy's, by Joe Wenderoth, was originally published by Wave Books in 2000.

"The Pajamaist," by Matthew Zapruder, originally appeared in the collection of the same name, published by Cooper Canyon in 2006.

Printed in the United States
by Baker & Taylor Publisher Services